BOOKS IN THE SPECIAL EDUCATION SERIES

SALLY M. ATACK is a graduate art teacher and a practicing artist with several years' experience in teaching the mentally and physically handicapped.

Art Activities
for the
Handicapped
A GUIDE FOR PARENTS AND TEACHERS

Sally M. Atack

additional material by
Mitylene Arnold, University of Georgia

A SPECTRUM BOOK

PRENTICE-HALL, INC., Englewood Cliffs, New Jersey 07632

Library of Congress Cataloging in Publication Data

ATACK, SALLY M.
  Art activities for the handicapped.

  "A Spectrum Book."
  Includes index.
  1. Handicapped children—Education—Art. I. Arnold,
Mitylene. II. Title.
LC4025.A85   1982   371.9′044   82-5282
ISBN 0-13-046995-5   AACR2
ISBN 0-13-046987-4 (pbk.)

10 9 8 7 6 5 4 3 2 1

Originally published in 1980 by Souvenir Press (Educational & Academic) Ltd., London, England, and
simultaneously in Canada. Copyright © 1980 by Sally M. Atack.

This Spectrum Book can be made available to businesses and organizations at a special discount when
ordered in large quantities. For more information, contact: Prentice-Hall, Inc., General Publishing Division, Special Sales, Englewood Cliffs, New Jersey 07632.

Cover design by Jeannette Jacobs
Cover illustration by April Blair Stewart
Manufacturing buyer: Cathie Lenard

ISBN 0-13-046995-5

ISBN 0-13-046987-4 {PBK}

Prentice-Hall International, Inc., *London*
Prentice-Hall of Australia Pty. Limited, *Sydney*
Prentice-Hall Canada Inc., *Toronto*
Prentice-Hall of India Private Limited, *New Delhi*
Prentice-Hall of Japan, Inc., *Tokyo*
Prentice-Hall of Southeast Asia Pte. Ltd., *Singapore*
Whitehall Books Limited, *Wellington, New Zealand*

Contents

III
CONCLUSION

IV
APPENDIXES

Preface

This book is primarily intended to help those working with mentally handicapped people, whether they are at home or in an educational or social setting. It may also be of interest to those working with young children. The aim of the book is to illustrate how drawing, painting, modeling, and making things can encourage development in children or adults with learning difficulties. As the book follows a developmental pattern, it is also relevant to the learning of young children. A number of ways in which art activities can assist development are explained, a pattern of development is explored, the provision and use of materials are discussed, and possible activities suggested.

This book arises out of practical experience with mentally handicapped children and young people (some of whom had additional handicaps), and also with physically handicapped children. However, it is beyond the scope of a book of this kind to suggest ways of helping all those with specific or multiple handicaps, as each child will present a unique problem.

Throughout this book I have addressed myself to the parents of children, often referring to "your child." This is not intended to exclude anyone but is done purely for simplicity. Actually, this book book will be useful not only to parents, teachers, classroom assistants, and nursery school aides or nurses, but also to those working in the field of continuing education and youth clubs for the handicapped. An interesting extension might encompass the many young people who are interested in voluntary work with handicapped individuals. They too might consider carrying out some of the suggestions.

Acknowledgments

I wish to acknowledge with thanks the contribution of the trainees and staff at New Malden Adult Training Centre, Surrey, England, without whom this book would not have been possible. I thank Dorothy Jeffree for help and encouragement; the children and staff at Meadow Court Special Unit for their help; Phil Hawks for his technical advice; Alice Sly and Laleah for typing the manuscript.

The photographs numbered 5.2, 5.3, 5.5, 5.10, 5.13, 6.5, and 6.7 were taken by Phillip Polglaze.

Art Activities
for the
Handicapped

I
INTRODUCTION TO ART ACTIVITIES

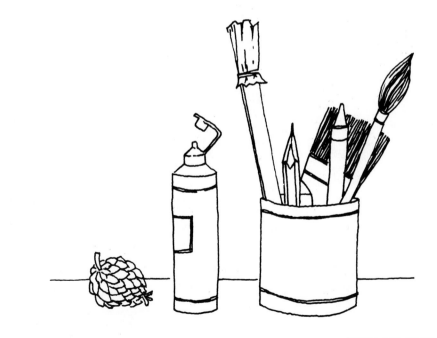

1

What Art Is and Does

WHAT IS ART?

In this book "art" is used as a loose term, and "art activities" should include all activities that involve the making of marks with, or in, almost any kind of material. The terms "painting" and "drawing" are intended to include daubs and scribbles as well as recognizable pictures, and the equivalent modeling terms to embrace simple squeezing and shaping of clay, as well as the building of models or pots.

This book intends to show how the artwork of children and maturing young people, whether they are handicapped or not, contains more than is immediately obvious. What we see is only the end product of a creative process. This process, the art of making a picture, is also a learning process and is at least as important as the picture itself. By watching and listening to children as they work, by providing facilities and materials appropriate to their needs, we can help them make the most of this learning.

Why Art at All?

It may not be easy to see how art activities can help a person develop. Probably few people would include the ability to draw or paint high on their list of essential survival skills. But have you ever noticed that when you come across something you don't instantly recognize or understand, you touch it or pick it up to find out more about it? It is no accident that gift shops display cards requesting people not to touch delicate articles, for shopkeepers have experienced our natural inclination to touch that which we like or find interesting, as well as that which we don't understand.

The exploration of things by touch is especially important to early development. Young children are naturally curious, and they pick things up and put them in their mouths to discover more about them. The joy of many elementary art activities for a child whose natural inclination to explore has been impaired is that they encourage this kind of exploration and discovery.

Art activities can be used to help the development of skills and abilities. Painting exercises can encourage the use and control of certain movements; art activities can stimulate the ability to organize oneself and one's thoughts; and organized group activities can develop cooperation and communication with others. But just as important, art activities give opportunities at all stages, and at all ages, to sink oneself in an activity for its own sake. There is no need for competition, for reward from other people, or even to have an end product in view. Art activities can simply be done for fun. They can be an outlet for emotion, and they add to the quality and variety of life. In this kind of activity a person is free to discover and explore, and much valuable learning takes place.

Many people today, and handicapped people in particular, find they have more and more leisure time. Instead of an opportunity for enriching their lives, this may mean only boredom and stagnation for young people who have not been shown ways of using their spare time well, in activities that extend them in new directions. Appropriately organized art activities may provide such an opportunity, combining pleasure and new learning.

HOW ART IS HELPFUL

Art can be helpful to people in a number of ways—by aiding in control and awareness of self; by building awareness and discrimination of things; by fostering communication; by strengthening contact with others; and by bringing pleasure and success.

Control and Awareness of Self

LEARNING TO MAKE SOMETHING
HAPPEN—PHYSICAL CONTROL

In the very early stages of physical development, actions are relatively uncontrolled. If you watch a very young baby, you will notice how many movements are relatively uncontrolled, many being reflex actions. Within the first few months of life, the child's control increases, and he or she differentiates particular movements. This is particularly obvious when a child first achieves the skill to grasp and then let go. The pleasure in practicing this new-found skill is clear in the baby who endlessly throws things out of the playpen, no matter how often they are picked up and returned.

In art activities it is possible to record the effect of other very simple physical actions. For example, moving a paint-covered hand across a piece of paper leaves a trail of paint marks on the paper. Pressing one's fingers into clay, or squeezing a lump of clay, leaves a visible and tactile impression. The pleasure of making marks in these ways can be as great as learning to "let go." There is a kind of magic in being able to make a mark. In this pleasurable activity, a child is not only learning to control his or her own movements, but is also discovering the subtleties of cause and effect, or the reasons why things happen. For some physically handicapped children who have limited opportunities to experience the effects of their own actions, simple art activities have a special value.

GETTING IT BETTER—
PHYSICAL DEXTERITY

Over a period of time (which may be a fairly lengthy period), a child will begin to control and direct his or her actions. With careful choice of art activities, you can encourage a child to use certain movements, and indicate that different movements make different sorts of marks. Gradually, instead of making random scribbled marks, the child will be able to choose to make particular marks, be they on clay or paper.

STRETCHING OUT—
THE PHYSICAL POSSIBILITY

Children can be presented with situations during art activities where they are, quite naturally, encouraged to explore their physical

5

limitations. Some activities will encourage the use and control of large movements, inviting children to stretch out, while others encourage the use of very small precise movements.

Awareness and Discrimination of Things

EXPLORING THE DIFFERENCE

Exploration has to do with discovering things, finding things out, by looking, touching, or doing. Exploration of some kind is tremendously important to learning at all stages of development. Art activities can give opportunity for several kinds of exploration. Particularly, in simple art activities children can be encouraged to learn, by handling materials of various characteristics, to become aware of differences in texture, shape, and size.

LEARNING THE DIFFERENCE

Growing from the physical exploration of things comes the ability to tell the differences between things, by looking as well as by touching. By selecting materials, and through conversational comment, such awareness can be reinforced. The ability to match two similar things by their shape, color, or size comes with the ability to tell the difference.

MAKING A CHOICE

Once a child has learned to tell the differences between things, he or she can begin to make choices. In the provision of materials, you can provide a child with simple opportunities to practice "telling the difference" and then to make choices. Very limited choice, among only two or three possibilities, should be offered to begin with so as not to confuse the child. Gradually the possibilities can be increased to include greater choice. Being free, and able, to make choices is an important personal liberty.

CHOOSING THE RIGHT THINGS—
PERSONAL ORGANIZATION

The developing child then progresses from making simple choices among two or three provided materials, to choosing and organizing for him- or herself several different materials required for a particular activity. Simple organizational habits can be established by storing art materials always in the same place and, if possible and practical, within easy reach. A child can then be directed toward finding and returning the required materials him- or herself.

MAKING CHOICES AND GETTING
THE RESULT—SELF-RELIANCE

Perhaps the final reward for a child comes with the personal satisfaction of knowing that he or she can make the necessary choices to achieve what was intended, and to "get it right"without reliance on others.

Communication

There is no doubt that the ability to communicate with others is of fundamental importance. As we usually use words to communicate, we tend to give that form of communication priority, but being able to talk is not the only way of communicating.

HAVING SOMETHING TO SHARE

Communication is a two-way thing. It is a process of sharing, and it needs two people giving and receiving. Just as a simple sound or cry is a form of communication, so too can be a simple mark on paper. Encourage this form of communication with your child, respond in a way the child can appreciate, perhaps with a smile or encouraging words.

ART AS LANGUAGE—A CONTACT
WITHOUT WORDS

It takes care on the part of the "teacher" or viewer of art to appreciate the full value of art as a form of communication. In the early stages, a child may tell most through the colors he or she chooses and the freedom with which he or she makes marks. As a child's ability to control those marks increases, the communicative value of his or her work also increases and the child will "tell" more about things, and him- or herself, through that art. Pictures will reflect those things a child finds most important and interesting. From the early stage, simply by showing care for a child's artwork, a valuable contact is established. Share the pleasure of art activities with your child whenever you can.

HAVING SOMETHING
TO TALK ABOUT

Because talking is the usual way in which we communicate with one another, it is also the most important way. Even though artwork can be a valuable form of communication in its own right, it can also be used as an inspiration for conversation. Having made a picture, a child has something rather special (special because the child has created it) that he or she may want to talk about. For those who do not talk about their work spontaneously, sensitive questions may encourage them to talk, but don't spoil the value of the nonverbal communication by insisting on the talk.

THIS IS HOW I SEE "IT"

As skill increases, the child is more and more able to give detailed views of how he or she sees things. The child can show in pictures the things he or she notices as being the most obvious or important. In your response you can demonstrate the value of that particular point of view, and thus express your value of the child as an individual.

PLACING A VALUE

A great deal of learning is achieved by copying an example. In setting an example, we encourage children to adopt similar values. In demonstrating your care for a child's work, you also demonstrate your care for that person. By this example, the child can learn to value his or her own work and that of others. A child can learn to be proud of personal achievements and sympathetic to the achievements of others.

As the growing interest in primitive art shows, the quality and value of a work of art does not depend upon technical know-how and sophisticated ideas, and certainly not on the measured intelligence of the artist. In this area, mentally handicapped people, given help, can sometimes come into their own and produce work that can be valued in its own right.

Contact with Others

JOINING IN

Art activities are noncompetitive activities in which people of all ages and abilities can join. It is inevitable that handicapped people are excluded from many activities because they lack the appropriate skills. Even though there are skills to be learned in art, it is an area of activity in which people of all ages and abilities can work alongside one another. Art is essentially an individual occupation; there is no score to be kept between opponents, no competition and no game to be won or lost. On the other hand the activity itself, the act of being occupied in the making of something, can be shared among several people.

SOMETHING TO GIVE

In making a drawing or a painting, a person is giving us a chance to see his or her point of view. This in itself is a kind of gift. The finished article too can be given away as a present. Only too often handicapped people find themselves "on the receiving end," with little opportunity to give to others. This places them in a very "unequal" situation, which would not help anyone's morale. Having something to give is of profound importance.

LETTING EXPERIENCE BE
THE BEGINNING OF ART

All art has to be about something. In the very early stages, it is likely to be about the experience of handling the materials and making simple marks. As progress is made, there are opportunities to make art activities relate to something outside that immediate experience and to some other aspect of the child's experience. Children can be encouraged to make pictures about things that have happened to them and about things that they have seen and found interesting.

Pleasure and Success

PLEASURE FROM HANDLING
MATERIALS

As already discussed, children gain pleasure simply from handling art materials—stirring and daubing, squeezing and squashing. This simple pleasure is something that more sophisticated artists continue to enjoy, and it is remarkable how many adults who return to art activities after a long break, perhaps since school days, comment on the soothing pleasure they find in simply handling materials.

PLEASURE FROM
HAVING MADE SOMETHING

Especially for the handicapped child, who has inevitably experienced failure in many other spheres, great satisfaction and enhanced self-esteem can be gained through having made something. Art activities can provide this opportunity. Remember that success needs to be acknowledged and can be reinforced by your response.

PLEASURE AND SUCCESS
FROM AN INTENDED RESULT

In the early stages of development, there may be no intention to make a particular thing, but as skills develop, a plan may be made. A child may plan to paint, say, a man, or to make a clay snake. A new pleasure can be gained from having successfully realized an intention.

PLEASURE THROUGH
BEING APPRECIATED

In appreciating a child's art, you demonstrate a care for him or her and the things the child enjoys in a special kind of way. This appreciation may at first be shown with a hug or a kiss, but can grow into an adult form of appreciation demonstrated by your continued care for the work.

PLEASURE THROUGH GIVING

Most people agree that as much pleasure is gained through giving as in receiving. A handicapped person may feel that he or she has not much to give, and thus has not experienced the joy of giving, but having made a picture, the person has something very special to give. Being able to give and to have your gift appreciated is of immeasurable value to all people, but particularly to the maturing young person.

2

Art Activity Stages
and Involvement

THE SIX DEVELOPMENT STAGES

The development stages in art activities follow a basic pattern, which is outlined below. Yet, as art activities rely upon perceptual, physical, and imaginative skills, all of which develop at different rates in different people, any individual child's development is inevitably uneven. You will notice periods of considerable activity and growth, and others of quiet consolidation.

The six development stages in art activities are:

Stage 1:
Discovery and Exploration

This is a time for free self-expression, a stage of experimenting and exploring. Materials should be used for fun. Activities at this stage are closely connected with the development of physical/motor skills, but also rely heavily upon the sensations, mainly felt through the fingers and hands.

Stage 2:
Discovering the Same Mark Again

At this stage an order is beginning to appear in the previously random work, and shapes made tend to be repeated. Development at this stage relies upon an increased control over physical movements so that marks are made with greater purpose, linked to an increased awareness of the differences between things and the ability to make simple choices.

Stage 3:
Making the Same Mark Again

Gradually, marks or shapes are made and more deliberately repeated; they may be remembered or copied from a previous occasion. At this stage the circle may have a particular importance. Patterns and objects a child makes will sometimes be given names. An increased awareness of similarity and differences develops, linked with greater physical control.

Stage 4:
Making Something Stand
For Something Else

Gradually the images become more recognizable and the links between the object or picture and the name given to it become clearer. At this stage, artwork can be a real source of conversation.

Stage 5:
Remembering the Past

With the ability to form a connection between images and real things, a child becomes able to make, and becomes interested in making, images about experiences outside of the art room. Although an event may be recorded or referred to in a picture, however, many apparent distortions will remain. Conversation and memory can play a very important role in image making at this stage.

Stage 6:
Seeing, Knowing, and Making

This is a stage when a child can make a fairly recognizable picture or model of something. Gradually heightened awareness enables him or her to "tell" us more about the things he or she sees. Although the child's work may still seem naive, it will have an air of considerable authority. A child's thinking will become more evident in the way he or she deliberately makes marks to stand for something.

WHAT ART ACTIVITIES INVOLVE

When we think of art, we tend to think of pictures or objects that are made to represent something recognizable, something we can enjoy looking at . . . and therein lies a trap! In considering the value of art activities, the finished drawing, painting, or model is not necessarily the most important thing. The finished piece has indeed a great deal of value, but the act of making has as much, or even more, at every level of attainment.

Too often teachers, both professional and other (see The Role of a Teacher in Chapter 3), are tempted to organize "art" activities for children that involve them in producing work bearing no relationship to the child's own developmental level. These activities are usually very well worked out, each child doing "his bit," exactly as told, and the final work put together by the teacher to create an impressive piece. These pictures have a superficial appeal, but they show a lack of respect for the children who "make" them, as neither the artistic impulse, nor the idea, nor the arrangement comes from the children. Each child must be respected for what he or she can do, at his or her own level.

Art activities should be used to encourage a child's development and to nurture real learning. To do this they must be provided at an appropriate level. Following are some guidelines.

1. The skills used in art activities follow a clear pattern of development. This is a natural pattern, closely related to other areas of maturity.

2. Art activities involve a process of learning, and work must be encouraged at an appropriate level. The right level can be found by observing the spontaneous gestures and marks made by a child (see Using This Book as a Guide, Chapter 4). Work at an inappropriate level will produce frustration or parrot-like mimicry without real understanding.

3. Each level of development has its own value and must be experienced fully before moving on to a more sophisticated stage. A vital part of learning may be missed if a stage is left out, thus further learning is hampered or inhibited completely.

4. The move from one level to another is a natural and gradual process. Following the pattern set out later in the book will help you prepare for and recognize the subtle changes between one stage and the next.

5. Each child will remain at any particular stage for a different length of time. There will be periods when no change is apparent, or even a backward move is observed. These are periods when learning is consolidated. There will also be periods when the level of an activity will not be maintained at its peak. Adults doodle to relieve boredom and a child's need to do something similar should be respected.

6. Everyone's final level of attainment is different. Many people will not reach the final stage of development, but they will be fulfilled by functioning happily and well at an earlier level.

3

You as Teacher

WHAT AND WHO IS A TEACHER?

A teacher is someone who enables other people to learn. A teacher is someone who can provide facilities and circumstances in which learning is as easy and as pleasurable as possible. But, when considering the role of a teacher, it is all too easy to think it necessary to impart information, to see ourselves as giving another the benefit of our own experience and expertise.

This kind of intervention can be very harmful to real learning unless supported by sensitive observation. Only through observation can we tell when to provide fresh opportunities for, or remove hindrances from, a pupil.

Don't be put off by the difficulties in the way of being a "good" teacher; anyone can take the role of teacher as this book envisages it, be they parent, friend, or helper, as well as the employed teacher. Everyone coming into contact with a handicapped person can contribute toward his or her growth. Parents are in a very good position to take the role of teacher, as they spend a great deal of time with their children and know them intimately.

THE ROLE OF A TEACHER

It is important to remember that when we adopt the role of teacher, we do take a very special role and one that has many different aspects. To help you understand the importance of this role, take note of the following roles of a teacher:

1. *As an observer.* This is one of the simplest roles of a teacher, but often one of the hardest to fulfill: it means simply to watch. Watching and remembering what a child does in particular circumstances often gives the vital clue to how to help a child most. It is only as a result of your observations that you will be able to provide for the individual needs of your child.

2. *As provider.* The teacher provides an appropriate space where art activities can take place without disruption. Time must also be made available, so that activities can be enjoyed without hurry. And, of course, materials must be provided according to the child's stage of development.

3. *As facilitator.* In the provision of suitable materials and space, the teacher can also become a facilitator. He or she can facilitate a simple process of choice and ease the development from one activity to another. Particularly for those suffering physical difficulties, your role is to make the activities as straightforward as possible, and even to adapt the activity and equipment to suit the individual need (see "It's Not as Easy as It Seems," Chapter 9).

4. *As an audience that cares.* For a child to enjoy and value artwork he or she creates, the child needs to feel that his or her contribution is of value. A demonstration of care for a child's artwork is very important to building up confidence. With confidence, a child will be encouraged to do more and perhaps better things.

4

Getting the Most
Out of Art Activities

Providing art activities can seem a daunting task, but simple organization can make the task easier. To make the most of any art activities, many things must be carefully considered, from selecting the right materials to keeping records of progress. This book can also be a helpful guide to getting the most out of art activities.

MATERIALS, SPACE, AND TIME

The ideas presented in Part II of this book cover a wide range of possible activities, but few of them require very special materials or equipment. Before buying materials, you should identify the level at which your child will be working, so as to decide on the most suitable materials for that stage. Activities are suggested in four main areas:

- Drawing.
- Painting.
- Cutting and pasting.
- Modeling.

The following materials form a basic list of equipment:

- Paper of various colors and sizes.
- Drawing equipment, such as pens, pencils, crayons, and felt pens.
- Paints of different consistencies.

- Brushes of various sizes.
- Scissors and paste.
- Clay or playdough.

Refer to the special list of materials in the particular section you use to find more information about appropriate materials before buying anything special. Throughout the suggested activities, you will find improvised equipment, for example, painting combs cut from cardboard, large "brushes" made from small pieces of sponge. Most of these ideas can be used without spending much extra money. (See Appendix B for information on art material suppliers.)

Whatever materials you use, clearly, almost any art activity is potentially messy, so it is essential to find a space where damage is least likely to be done to walls, floors, or furniture. A table with a wipe-clean top placed in a uncarpeted room would be ideal, but may not be possible. Newspaper can offer some protection from paints and crayons, but is not much good when using clay or playdough. Large plastic sheets can be bought cheaply to protect tables, floors, and even walls from paint or clay splashes, but remember that plastic can make a slippery surface on the floor or table. When using clay or playdough, a wooden board like a cutting or pastry board works well, as does a piece of plywood placed on the table. The bare wood has a slightly absorbent surface so that the clay or playdough will not stick in the way that it would to plastic. Good organization saves valuable energy and time, so accept the limitations of space and work within them.

From both parent's and child's point of view, it is important that art activities be attempted only where fear of damage is minimal. Anxiety felt by either would be detrimental to the success of the activity.

Anxiety about time can also be detrimental. Time is a surprisingly important factor in the success of art activities. Not only is it important for children to have sufficient time to enjoy an activity, but it is also necessary to have enough time to clear away the mess at the end without feeling pressured. Art activities should be pleasurable and can be spoiled by feeling rushed.

Every child will be interested in a single project for a different length of time, and you will learn with experience how long your child's interest will last.

Routine is often important to young children, whether they are handicapped or not, but as we can all recall from our own school days we do not always feel like "doing art" on a particular day, or at a particular time of day, just because it is the established routine. Therefore, when choosing a time for art, remain sensitive both to the need for routine and to the child's desire to take part.

When organizing a routine and providing materials, remember that simple drawing activities can be provided for with little preparation and can be available at almost any time. It is important that a child have freedom to use drawing materials as much as possible, even when you are unable to join in. Yet don't let a child's willingness to entertain him- or herself with drawing persuade you to withdraw. Your interest and involvement are very valuable and should be freely given.

OTHER CONSIDERATIONS

Variety

When choosing and organizing activities for your child, it is important to include elements of both repetition and variety. Don't be afraid to repeat the same thing several times; the repetition of known activities can be very positive, as it reinforces learning and builds confidence. But a variety of activities can help a child to use established skills in alternative settings. The transfer of learning from one situation to another can be assisted by the use of two or three different activities with similar skills.

The introductions to the activities in Part II of this book will help you in your choice, but simple variations can be achieved by providing a slightly different choice of materials for the same activity. Playdough can be used as an alternative to clay; the color of paper and paints can be varied and drawings can be encouraged in pencil crayon as a change from wax crayons. These slight variations have special importance to children who need a lot of encouragement to move from one developmental stage to another; variation will help to keep and stimulate their interest.

The development from one stage to another will be a slow process, and it is a good idea to adapt known activities so that they become gradually more sophisticated without disrupting an established pattern of activity too much. Guided by the introductions to the chapters in Part II, try your own variations. Remember that the ideas offered are only suggestions.

Exhibitions

One of the pleasures of art activities is that something is made as a result of them. Although the finished work is not necessarily the most important part of the activity, and valuable learning takes place along the way, the finished work does have importance. A piece of artwork is something that can be looked at and admired. Make the most of this value by creating an exhibition. Perhaps wall space could be put aside for the display of pictures and suitable space made for three-dimensional artwork on a shelf or the top of a low bookcase, but essentially where the child will be able to see his or her own work. It is even more important for the child to see his or her own work than it is for you to be able to see and admire it.

Displaying something means that it can be seen over and over again, and this may be important in a child's development. Not only can a child grow in self-respect through being appreciated, but the child may learn by looking at the results of his or her own efforts. The very fact that a picture is there to be seen may be sufficient to alter a child's view of his or her own work. The actual looking does not *need* to be directed, but thoughtful directions may help in an objective view of the work. Simply by looking and comparing, a child may be able to recognize what is happening in his or her drawings and strive to "do it again," or to put a special kind of effort into another piece. This recognition can happen even at an early stage, when scribbles begin to show a sense of order, or when the first shapes are repeated. Unless the pictures are displayed so that they can be seen again and again, a child has little opportunity to reflect upon the results of his or her efforts, or fully to appreciate what he or she has done.

Records

The changes in a child's artwork are often quite subtle and will rarely be noticeable from one day to another. To build a diary or history of development, it is a good idea to keep the work done by your child. It is from an overview of a number of pieces of work that any development will become apparent. This is particularly important when looking for hints indicating a move from one stage to another. Always date the work and, if working with more than one child, add the child's name. The date really is *most* important; there is nothing more frustrating than reviewing a large selection of work and being unable to remember the sequence.

Papers are fairly easy to store; they can be placed flat in folders made from heavy cardboard (perhaps the sides of very large cardboard cartons) and stored against a wall or under a bed. Three-dimensional work is more difficult to store. Small quantities can be kept in cardboard boxes. Should the quantity become so great that it is essential to throw some away, make sure that you look at the collected work as a continuing record from earliest work, and discard only work that is clearly similar to work retained. This is best done when signs of progress have become visible. Always retain a body of work representative of every stage. Not only does this act as a guide to the provision of activities, but it will become a rewarding record of progress.

USING THIS BOOK AS A GUIDE

Finding the Right Level

Before thinking about organizing an activity for your child, it is important to discover the level at which he or she is functioning. It is essential to find the real level of ability your child has reached before providing an activity. This may sound both obvious and easy, but it is all too easy to be biased in a judgment by a child's social behavior—that is, how he or she behaves in company with other people. This may be more competent, or less, than the child's ability to express him- or herself creatively. There is no point in encouraging children to do complex things until they are really confident in simple tasks. I can only stress the importance of each level of learning and that the skills at each level must be experienced and thoroughly learned before moving to the next level.

Discovering the actual level of achievement of a child involves watching the way in which he or she does things when not being directed or helped. These spontaneous actions may best be observed when your child is in a familiar situation, or one where he or she has to make no choices. It may, therefore, be easier to see the clues while your child is playing or eating than when using crayons or paints. Watch what your child does when using a spoon to eat with; does he or she bang the spoon up and down, or stir the food? Or see what sort of marks or patterns your child will make on a steamed-up mirror or window.

The chart that follows suggests possible things to look out for in various situations, and relates these to the appropriate stage of art activities described later in this book.

FINDING THE RIGHT LEVEL OF WORK

DEVELOPMENTAL STAGE	CHAPTER IN THIS BOOK	ACTIONS TO LOOK FOR
Before Stage 1		Grips, but cannot release at will.
		Explores objects habitually by putting them into the mouth.
Stage 1: Discovery and exploration	Chapter 5	Grips, opens, and closes hands at will.
Stage 2: Discovering the same mark again		Bangs spoon up and down.
		Stirs food from side to side or in circles.
		Makes archlike pattern or circles in steamed-up mirror or soft sand, etc.
		Usually eats food with fingers.
Stage 3: Making the same mark again	Chapter 6	Habitually makes circle patterns or shapes:
Stage 4: Making something stand for something else		$\mathcal{C}$
		Can follow a down line with finger.
		Usually eats food with a spoon.
		Recognizes generally similarities between two objects or pictures.
Stage 5: Remembering the past	Chapter 7	Attempts to draw objects or people without prompting.
		Has a good recall of things that have happened in the past.
Stage 6: Seeing, knowing, and making	Chapter 8	Makes recognizable drawings of things he or she can see.
		Notices details about what makes two similar objects different.

Knowing the Book

Chapters 5, 6, 7, and 8 in Part II of this book represent levels of attainment as shown in the chart. Each chapter contains suggested activities appropriate to the level of development described.

After having established, with the help of the chart, the level of development your child has reached, read the introduction to the chapter indicated. Unless the introduction seems to suggest that the activities are too advanced for your child, start by choosing from the ideas an activity you think will appeal to your child. Don't be afraid to begin with very basic activities, even those described in a chapter before the one indicated; your child will quickly show you if he or she has greater skills.

Browse through the entire book before you start, to get the feel of how activities can be developed. Although the appropriate chapter can be found without reading the text, being familiar with the whole book places each activity into the context of overall development. Some of the suggestions made in alternative chapters may also help you to develop new and different ideas.

Points to Remember

Before beginning the activities, here are some points to remember:

- *Try your own variations.* The activities offered are only suggestions; try out some of your own ideas.
- *Repeat the same activity.* Repetition is a way of establishing new learning. Once the learning is established, your child will probably instigate a change in the activity him- or herself.
- *Limit the possibilities.* Particularly in the early stages, limit the number of alternatives available so as not to cause confusion and frustration.
- *Observe rather than lead.* Try to take a lead from your child, observing natural reactions to the activities you provide, and make other activities available to use and encourage skills.
- *All things take time.* Don't try too much too soon. All new learning takes time. There is often a period of rest or even of slight regression after a period of new learning.
- *All people develop differently.* Each person develops at a different rate and in different directions from another. Don't expect two children to react the same way to any given activity.
- *A shared problem is a problem lessened.* Try to find a friend with whom to compare notes and share problems. It is always useful to have someone to talk to about difficulties and *successes*.
- *Avoid a choice between working or wrecking.* Avoid situations allowing bad or destructive behavior. If a child behaves destructively, remove the activity and

try it at a later date. If necessary, attempt an alternative activity on the next occasion. Should these attempts be unsuccessful, try to find a totally different activity in which your child finds greater pleasure and fulfillment.

- *Enjoy yourself.* Above all, art activities should be enjoyable. Make them as pleasurable and stress-free as possible for your children.

II

ACTIVITIES
FOR STAGES
OF DEVELOPMENT

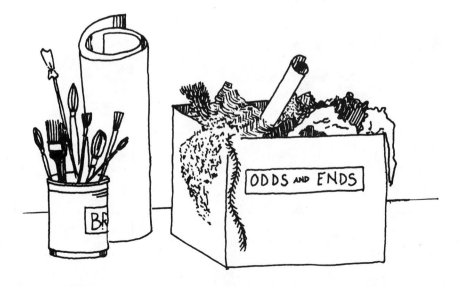

5

Activities for Stages 1 and 2

STAGE 1: DISCOVERY
AND EXPLORATION

STAGE 2: DISCOVERING THE
SAME MARK AGAIN

The first two development stages are covered together because the links between them are very strong and the suitable activities will be largely the same for both. Also explored are some ways of extending the activities, and you will no doubt find other ways of developing them yourself.

The activities in this chapter are designed for the very young child and for those who have acquired little control over their physical movements. "Children who have little control" refers to those whose natural tendency is to make large swinging movements with their hands and arms, not tiny or refined movements using subtle wrist and finger actions. The activities rely upon the "here and now" and make little or no reference to past experience, as children functioning at this stage also have limited powers of recall.

The work suggested in this chapter is to encourage exploration of and discoveries about materials, and about the simple movements the child can make. The activities are designed to encourage control of physical actions, to increase strength, and to encourage visual and tactile awareness. These together form an essential basis upon which greater skills and achievements can be built. Most of the work in this chapter will be messy or "scribbly," so be prepared.

GENERAL HINTS

LIMIT THE POSSIBILITIES

This is a stage for finding out what happens, how things feel and what they look like, a time for exploring and a time for discovering. At a time like this, when most of the experiences you are providing are new, it is important to limit the possibilities so that the child does not become overwhelmed and confused. Discovery is itself a kind of learning, and we want to make the learning as easy as possible. Tackle only one activity in any one session and limit the alternatives within the activity.

The range of colors available at this stage would best be restricted to the primaries—red, yellow, and blue; all good, clear, bright colors, and a range that can be added to later. If using clay, limit the possibilities, for example, by limiting the number of objects for pressing into clay to three or four, so that the child can easily appreciate what is happening, but has enough variety to retain interest.

It may be a surprise to you, if you work out the total possible combinations among only three colors, to see how many possibilities you are offering a child at any one time. Work it out and then ask yourself whether you could remember the same number of new facts at one sitting? In this way, the simple tasks we present to our children are put into a more realistic perspective.

HERE AND NOW

All the activities in this chapter are concerned only with what is happening at the time of the activity. They do not make reference to things that cannot be seen or to occasions that are past. They are essentially to do with the "here and now."

Of course, it may be possible to begin to make links with the past, particularly in a subsequent session of the same activities. It will be possible to draw your child's attention to such things as colors, textures, and even shapes in other situations as well as during art activities. This will inevitably help learning to take place.

MAKE THE MOST OF MOVEMENT

Most of the movements made by children functioning at this early stage will be big movements, so make the most of them. Don't be afraid to encourage sweeping actions. They are quite natural, and it is only through gradually learning to control the large movements that finer control grows.

DON'T USE TOO MUCH TIME

A child's concentration span is often quite short, so it is important to make the most of it, but not to attempt to continue after interest has gone. The span of concentrated effort will naturally grow.

DON'T EXPECT TOO MUCH

Don't expect to see developments within weeks. Small changes will take place, but developments are likely to show clearly only after a long period of activity. This is why it is so important to keep work as a record (see Chapter 4 under Other Considerations).

REPETITION

Don't be afraid to repeat activities. It is very important for a child to discover the same thing over and over again, so that he or she really remembers it and learns.

SHARING AND GIVING

As always, parents, friends, and teachers have a very special role to play in their willingness to share the pleasure of an activity, and in appreciating the end product.

JOINING IN AND ENJOYING YOURSELF

There are many opportunities for you to join in the art activities, even at this early stage. To make it easier, think of the activities as a kind of game; play with your child and enjoy yourself.

THINGS TO DO
Getting the Feel of It

It is through our sense of touch that much early discovery and learning occurs. Our lips and tongues are undoubtedly the most sensitive parts of our bodies, and it is no accident that very young children pick things up and put them in their mouths. But our hands, and particularly our fingers, are also very sensitive.

FINGER PAINTING

Finger painting gives children the opportunity to "squish" around as they might in mud or wet sand; a kind of playing that comes naturally to most children and plays an important part in their development. Finger painting is not only a slightly more sophisticated way of offering this form of exploration, and somewhat less messy and more acceptable indoors, but the paints are colored. At the end of the activity, you have a picture to keep as a permanent record.

To begin with, the fact that the paints are colored may not appear to be important to the child. He or she may treat them indiscriminately. It will become important as soon as the child notices the differences between them.

The finished painting in any case provides a permanent record of the movements that made it. It is something to keep and look at again.

Paints and paper.   All that is needed for finger painting is a large piece of paper and jars of ready mixed paints. Commercial finger paints can be expensive, so make your own by mixing cold water paste with poster paints to make a thick paint that a child can spread easily with hands or fingers. If your child is able to help him- or herself to paint, try to find jars that have large enough tops to dip fingers in (see Figure 5.1).

Remember that any two primary colors mixed together make a third color, and that all three primary colors mixed make brown or gray.

Use a large sheet of paper. It is a good idea to attach the paper to the table with masking tape so that it does not move around.

Show that it's all right.   Sometimes it is difficult to engage a child in finger painting, particularly if he or she has been taught to keep clean while playing. Older mentally handicapped people also are often reluctant to join in at first. It is, therefore, important to demonstrate that it is all right to mess with paints and that the

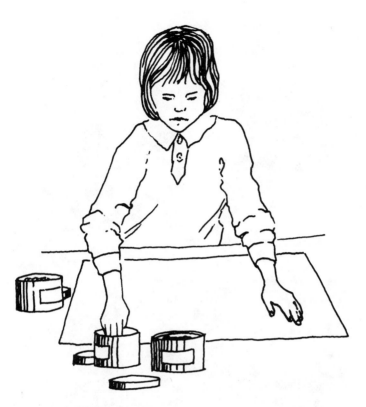

FIGURE 5.1. Scraping finger paints from a jar.

children won't get "told off" for getting their clothes dirty. It helps to join in yourself to show that it really is acceptable. Be sure to provide appropriate covering for the arms and body. Ideally, washing facilities should be close by so that hands, arms, and faces can be quickly cleaned up. Even where washing facilities are near, have a damp sponge ready for emergencies. A child may be quite happy to experiment without help, and that is fine, but there are some things that you might usefully encourage your child to do.

Reaching and spreading. Encourage work on quite large pieces of paper, so that a child has to stretch to reach the top. (Although we refer to the "top" of a painting, don't be upset if a child walks around the painting, or turns the painting around, so that he or she works from all sides. This is quite natural, and may indeed encourage more stretching and reaching.)

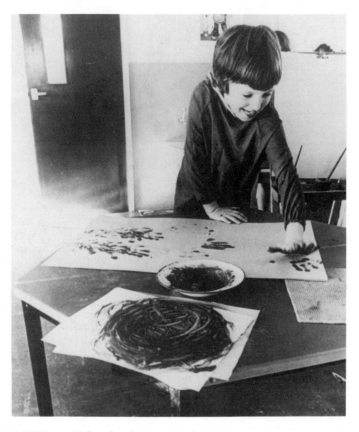

FIGURE 5.2. Making hand prints—reaching out.

REACHING OUT—
MAKING HAND PRINTS

Children often enjoy simply making hand prints on paper (see Figure 5.2). Encourage your child to reach out and fill empty spaces, or to experiment with making several prints one on top of another. Make it into a game in which you can join. Try making hand prints when the paper is flat on the table, at an easel, or even stuck on the wall.

MAKING CIRCLES

It is important for a child to make the kind of exploratory movements that come most naturally. They may be banging, up-and-down movements, or side-to-side rubbing movements. It can also be helpful to aid a child in the discovery of new movements. Try demonstrating different movements, or take your child's hands and

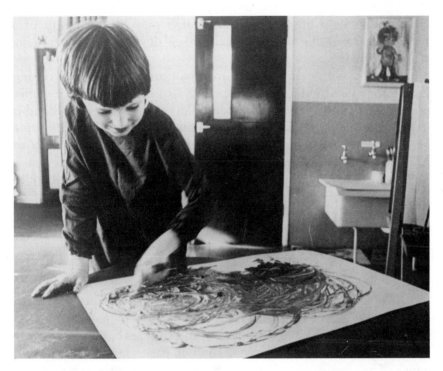
FIGURE 5.3. Finger painting—making circles.

make him or her feel new movements. Encourage a rhythmic side-to-side arch movement and large circular movements (see Figure 5.3).

SPREADING AND MIXING

In the very early stages, children may pay no attention to the colors that they are using, and simply mix them together without noticing their differences. Encourage a child's awareness of the colors he or she is using by comparing them with other things you can see, and draw attention to how the colors change when they are mixed together.

Talk about what is happening, and join in some of the time.

SCRIBBLING

Long before it is possible to make a recognizable picture, a child must get the feel of holding a pencil or crayon. Scribbling is one of the very first kinds of mark a child will make, but as soon as he or she is able to hold a pencil or crayon and bring it down on a table top, a child can make a mark. The first marks may be the result of a banging action, but with practice these will develop into continuous scribble.

As in finger painting, children will probably begin working with either hand with equal happiness. But it is unusual for someone to continue this practice when holding a pencil, as one hand is usually far more comfortable to use than the other. (There are some exceptions to this; some people, known as ambidextrous, use both hands with equal ease.) Notice which hand your child uses habitually and encourage him or her to use mostly that hand. Be careful not to force the use of the right hand only, however, unless your child indicates clearly that it is the more comfortable, since he or she may be a naturally left-handed person. Bear in mind also that your child may want to experiment, even at a later stage, using both hands to draw or paint, to see what it feels like, or to see the effect it has on the work.

It is a good idea to secure a sheet of paper to the table with masking tape, until your child is able to hold it still him- or herself. It is also advisable to provide a fairly strong paper, as children are likely to draw with considerable vigor and will easily make holes in thin paper. This can prove very disappointing and cause considerable upset, so it is better avoided.

Give guidance.   If a child finds difficulties making a continuous scribble mark, guide his or her hand to demonstrate the kind of movements it is possible to make and help him or her get the feel of it. The natural movements will be large swinging movements with a bending movement at the elbow, or even a swing from the shoulder.

Stretching up.   Encourage your child to stretch and scribble as far as possible, using paper on a table top. For full arm movements, put the paper on a wall or a board placed almost vertically.

JOIN IN AND PLAY GAMES
A child will probably be encouraged by your "joining in." Try working on a sheet next to the child's rather than on the same one, perhaps demonstrating the kind of marks you make using the characteristic arm swinging movements. Invent other scribbling games that you can both play on the same or different sheets. Most of these games will involve mimicry, such as "can you reach as high as this?" or "can you make a mark like this?" It is essential to watch what your

child does naturally and invent your games to exploit the skills of control and awareness he or she has acquired. Base all your games on things you know your child can do, and help him or her to get better at them. Stretching games encourage the ability to reach out or up, copying games encourage greater control, and both encourage greater awareness both of the child and of his or her work.

Encourage the making of circles.   As the child becomes more familiar with scribbling, encourage him or her in your games to make circular movements, to draw shapes that resemble circles or ovals. Not only do these shapes usually take on a particular significance at a later stage of development, but they also encourage movements of the wrist and elbow.

Vary the choice of materials.   A pencil may seem rather ordinary to scribble with, so have available other materials; wax crayons and felt pens are both good, as they have thick points and come in bright colors. Don't be afraid to extend the scribbling activities to include painting with large brushes (see Figure 5.4), but be prepared for the mess. Again, don't prolong the activity if interest is flagging.

Making connections with colors.   Even at this early stage of color use, it is possible to draw connections between the colors being used and those that can be seen around you. Point out colors on the child's clothes or in the room. Because it is difficult for the child to remember, it is not usually helpful to make connections with things that are not visible.

Making connections with shapes.   It can be useful to talk about the kinds of marks that appear in the scribbles your child makes, encouraging him or her to compare the shapes he or she has drawn with the shapes of things he or she can see. This becomes easier once enclosed shapes, such as circles or ovals, appear. Children tend to become more willing to name things when they can draw them, which is itself a developmental step. It is important to give a child the opportunity to make his or her own connections between the marks he or she makes and the things he or she knows, so be sympathetic to a child's stage of development when making comparisons, and go at the child's pace. The child who has difficulties with language may be reluctant or unable to make verbal connections, however, so may need to be prompted and helped.

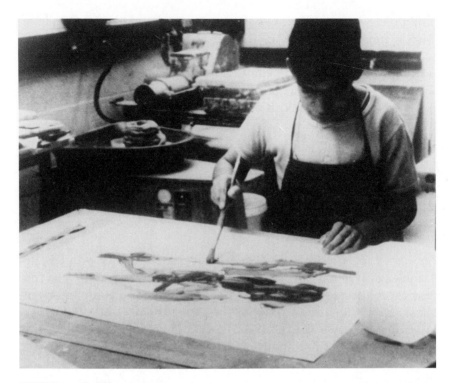

FIGURE 5.4. Scribble painting.

SQUEEZING, SQUASHING, PINCHING, AND PRODDING

Clay or playdough provide marvelous opportunities for exploration and discovery, and also encourage movements of hands and fingers (see Figure 5.5). Both materials, but clay in particular, have a satisfying texture that invites touching, pressing, squeezing, and squashing (see Appendix A). Further, clay can provide a range of tactile experiences: it can be used in its usual malleable plastic state, when cheese-hard, and even when it is wet and sticky or hard and brittle. It must be remembered that the greatest benefit of work at this stage is in its contribution to a child's exploration and learning through the use of materials. At this stage of all stages, the end result has least significance.

Like finger painting, work with clay may prove difficult with those afraid of getting dirty. The problem is greater when using the red- or brown-colored clay rather than the gray. If you meet with resistance, coax carefully and use gray clay in preference to red.

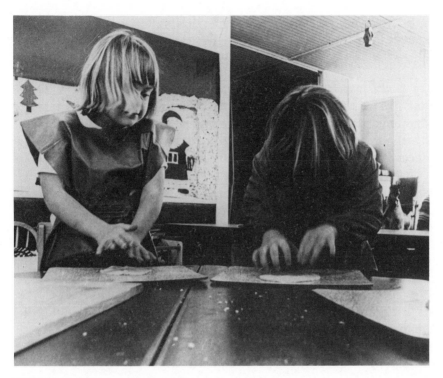

FIGURE 5.5. Poking, prodding, and patting clay.

Malleable clay. Work with clay in its usual malleable state should be done on an unvarnished wooden surface (an old cutting or pastry board will do, but not a plastic-coated one), or on a heavy closely woven cloth, such as canvas. The clay is damp, so it will inevitably stick slightly to any surface, but the mildly absorbent nature of wood or canvas reduces this tendency considerably. If you use cloth, secure it to a heavy board or to the table to prevent it moving around.

The amount of clay that you offer a child will in some way affect what he or she does, so experiment and watch what happens. To begin with, you might provide a piece of clay large enough to be held in both hands (the hands of the child); that is, not too big to get hold of and yet not so small that you can't do anything with it. Simply picking up the ball of clay and holding it in one or both hands uses the strength of fingers, hands, and wrist, and can be the beginning of a more thorough exploration. Gently encourage your child to discover what can be done to clay by poking, prodding, squeezing, and squashing. Don't be disappointed if this is all you achieve for some time, for these little experiments form the basis of a better understanding and encourage valuable movements.

Try smaller pieces.   Try also small pieces of clay that have to be pinched, torn, or broken from the main lump. To begin, do this for your child, demonstrating how it is done, but don't forget to encourage those who are strong enough to try for themselves. Smaller pieces of clay can be squashed in one hand or between two; they can be flattened with the fist or rolled under the hand along the table (see Figure 5.6). Encourage as far as you can the simple handling of clay so that your child learns how clay behaves and what he or she can do with it. Enjoy with the child such things as the pleasure of squeezing clay in a tightly held fist, and the surprise of the resulting intriguing shape.

Wet and sticky clay.   It may not be appropriate at first to offer clay in its alternative states, and particularly not wet and sticky clay, to children who are afraid of getting dirty. But once it seems appropriate and possible, offer children opportunities to enjoy and explore the squidgy, squelchy properties of wet clay.

FIGURE 5.6. Rolling and pressing patterns into clay.

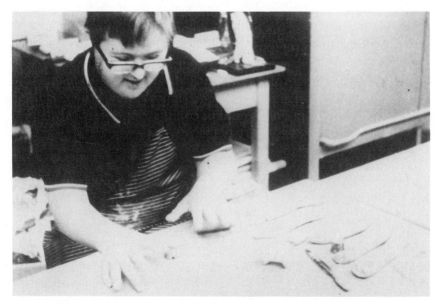

Work with wet clay is obviously going to be messy so be prepared. Remember that there is a time in the cycle of the reconstitution of clay when it has to be moistened and made sticky, and then dried out. This may be an appropriate opportunity to offer this alternative as part of the activity.

Dry clay.   It may be necessary to reserve the use of cheese-hard and dry clay until children have greater control of physical skills. Tools are necessary in the cutting and shaping of hardening clay, and in the scraping and scoring of brittle clay. Both require good physical control and well-directed strength.

Make Something Happen

We make something happen in all art activities, but comb painting and squeezy painting are special.

COMB PAINTING

Comb painting is not only fun to do, but the effect produced at the time is interesting; also there are additional discoveries to be made when the picture is dry. This is a good method to use with children who can grip and control large tools, but still rely on large swinging movements of the hands and arms. Large cardboard combs are used instead of paintbrushes.

How to make a comb.   Combs used for painting are made from cardboard. Since the combs get wet, try to use thick cardboard so that they can be used as long as possible. Cardboard that soaks through too easily will bend and is of no use. The back of a note pad will probably be thick enough. Cut the combs as illustrated in Figure 5.7, making several broad teeth with fairly large spaces in between. The size of the teeth and the spaces between them can be varied as you wish. The piece of card above the teeth should be nice and broad to give the child plenty to grip.

Mixing the paint.   Comb pictures are best made with thick paint, so finger paints can be used, but home-mixed paints can be as good. Mix acrylic glue or "gesso" with water-based paints to make a fairly stiff consistency. It must be stiff enough to stand up in small ridges without melting away, but thin enough to spread with ease. Use only two colors to begin with.

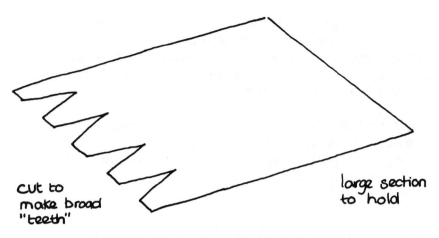

cut to
make broad
"teeth"

large section
to hold

FIGURE 5.7. How to make a cardboard painting comb.

Using the comb.   Have a large sheet of fairly substantial paper to work on. The paper must be quite strong as it will get fairly wet also. Spoon a quantity of prepared paint onto the paper. Using the comb like a large brush, the child can spread the paint around. The teeth will scrape the paint across the paper, leaving only a thin layer, while much more paint will remain in grooves where the spaces between the teeth have passed. The marks left are a series of gaps and ridges similar to those made with the fingers in finger painting (see Figure 5.8).

Making patterns.   It may be necessary at first to demonstrate and guide your child in the use of the comb. The child will probably find it easier to use it standing up than sitting down, but will probably need your hand guiding his or hers to begin with. Once the child has the hang of it, encourage him or her to experiment with the kinds of patterns he or she can make, making lines overlap or cross over one another. Start with one color so that the effect of the comb can be clearly understood. Later introduce the second color, which may serve to stimulate a new kind of exploration relating to the mixing of the colors as well as to the ridge patterns.

Exploring the dry picture.   Allow the painting to dry out completely. As it does, the glue will harden and the ridges will become permanent. The finished effect is best appreciated by the sense of touch, not just by looking. Show your child how to feel the ridges by running his or her hand over them. Remind the child that he or she made the ridges

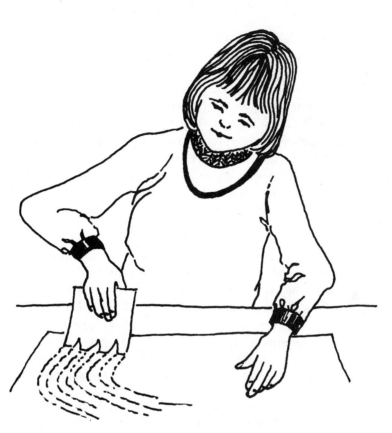

FIGURE 5.8. Using a cardboard painting comb.

by painting with a comb. It is important that the link between the wet and the dry painting is understood by your child, as it may have an important effect on subsequent work. It may be a good idea on subsequent occasions to explore a dried comb painting before making another.

Explore other textures. Having explored the texture of the picture, you may be able to find other things around you that have ridge patterns or textures, such as corduroy, cane chair seats, or even the child's own clay work, for your child to feel and compare with his or her picture. Let this become a game of discovering new textures.

SQUEEZY PAINTING
This method of making marks can be great fun. It requires and encourages the use of strong hands and arms; the arms to lift and direct, the hands to squeeze.

Mixing the paint. As the paints are to be squeezed from plastic bottles, they must be mixed to a fairly thick, but runny, consistency. Mix water-based paints with acrylic glue, gesso, or water paste. Ready-mix paints can be bought already mixed to about the right consistency, but they are fairly expensive. Mix colors either with acrylic glues or cold water paste. If acrylic glue is added as the main mixing medium, the paint will dry with a lovely, glossy, plastic finish. Although adding acrylics could also prove expensive if repeated often, the results are sufficiently interesting to look at, to feel, and talk about to make it worth trying once in a while. The shiny surface produced is a good one to compare with the roughness of comb paintings (see earlier this section).

Squeezy bottles. Put different colors into empty dishwashing liquid bottles and replace the tops. (You may have to use a funnel to get the paint into the bottle.) Since the bottles are not transparent, it is useful to indicate the color by labeling them with paper of the appropriate color. You might put a protective layer of transparent, self-adhesive tape over the paper on bottles you intend to use on several occasions. Household paints can be used to mark the bottles, but they tend to flake off when the bottle is squeezed.

Making the picture. The painting will be heavy because the layer of paint will be so thick, so provide a large piece of strong paper or thin cardboard. The paint can be applied to the paper right from the bottle, so make sure your child sits or stands high enough above the paper to be able to manipulate the bottle. It is best for children to stand or kneel on a chair at a table, or alternatively to work on the floor, kneeling or standing up.

Trailing the paint. Show your child how to squeeze the paint from the bottle and encourage him or her to direct the flow of paint around the paper (see Figure 5.9). Allow the child to explore the possibilities of this activity, learning how to control the flow of paint. Encourage him or her to direct the marks he or she makes. To increase awareness of where the marks are being made, have two or three colors available so he or she can make contrasting color areas.

Altering the trailed picture. There is no need for brushes with this method of making marks. The squiggly-squirly marks can be left as they are. Yet, as a variation, the paint applied in this way can be moved about either with brushes or with wide cardboard spatulas.

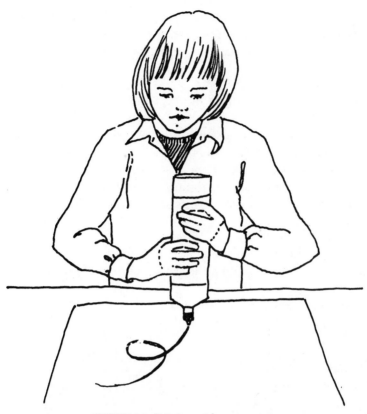

FIGURE 5.9. Painting with squeezy paints.

Reaching Out

All the activities in this chapter so far involve children in a certain amount of stretching and reaching, but some activities can be designed especially to help a child reach farther than usual. In drawing and painting activities, we naturally extend our reach by using a paintbrush or pencil, and there are many ways in which children can be encouraged to use these tools to stretch out even farther.

STANDING AND WALKING
AROUND A PICTURE

Some children choose to stand while they are drawing or painting; this increases their range and also enables them to paint from all sides of the picture. Painting from all sides is quite natural at this stage; it is much later in development that images begin to appear the "right way up." Children are quite likely to draw upside down as well as right way up even when they begin drawing recognizable images. Encourage children who are reluctant to stand to kneel on their chairs so that they too can reach farther.

SPONGES ON STICKS

As an alternative to ordinary paintbrushes, try makeshift brushes by attaching pieces of sponge or rag to the end of pieces of stick. The handles or sticks can be any length you choose, and this makes them particularly good for making floor paintings. To increase a child's awareness of the distance he or she can reach, try beginning a painting using ordinary brushes and then extend the scope of the work with the introduction of the sponge brushes.

SPONGE PAINTING

Sponges themselves can be a substitute for paintbrushes, and may prove easier for some children to use (see Figure 5.10). The

FIGURE 5.10. Painting with a sponge—enjoying the dribbles.

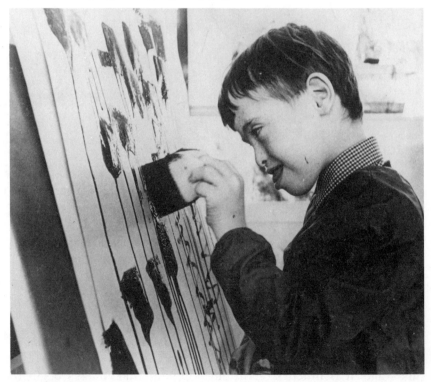

range of marks made by others may be greatly extended with the addition of sponges. Experiment with the size you give to the children. Sometimes put the paper on a table, sometimes on the floor, and sometimes at an easel or on the wall (see Figure 5.11). Encourage stretching games as before.

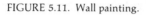

FIGURE 5.11. Wall painting.

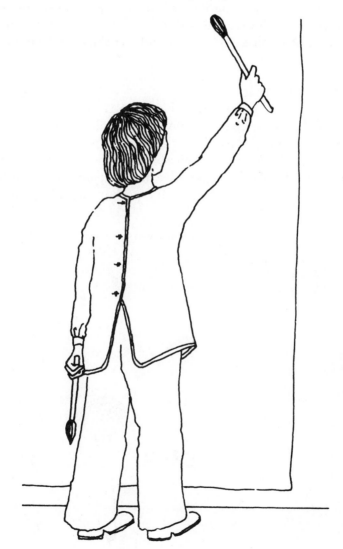

WALL PAINTING

A large sheet of paper hung on a wall provides a good surface on which to play stretching games. Stick several sheets of paper together, if necessary, to make a sheet as large as possible. Children can be encouraged to reach both upward and sideways, and this is best done standing up. If the space is large enough, encourage the most extravagant movements to illustrate to a child the vast space that can be covered by stretching the arms without moving the feet. Experiment. Encourage marks made in different ways, from simple hand prints and paint trailed with the fingers, to marks made with ordinary paintbrushes (or household brushes) and sponges on sticks.

FLOOR PAINTING

Painting on the floor (see Figure 5.12) can also encourage children to be more than usually mobile, although this may be difficult to arrange. I have done this kind of painting outside on a fine day, but problems arise when a breeze blows up. One advantage of the increased scale that is possible in floor painting is that two or more children can join in the activity, perhaps learning from each

FIGURE 5.12. Floor painting with sponges on sticks.

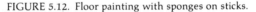
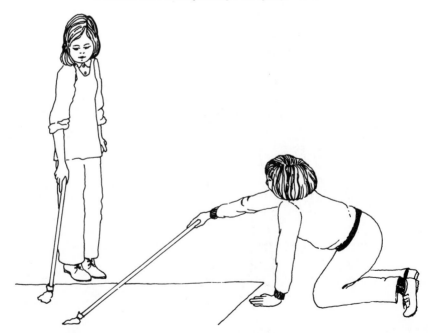

other, without necessarily interfering with each other's marks. The whole painting could be put on the wall when dry. Children can be encouraged to look at, point to, and reach the marks that interest them.

Choosing and Arranging

In most art activities some choice is given. In the early stages it is best to keep choices to a minimum so as not to confuse the child. The following activities deliberately offer choices and encourage simple decision making. They are specifically designed to encourage choices about where a mark will be made.

POTATO OR SPONGE PRINTS
You do not make fancy potato cuts at this stage, but use cut potatoes simply as mark makers. It is easy to hold half a potato and put it down on paper. So it is possible to make a very simple mark or print simply by first dipping the cut side in paint.

You may have other and better ideas as to what can be used to make prints in this way (see Figure 5.13). I have used pieces of firm sponge designed as pan cleaners (they have a hard scratchy side useful for holding), and have also experimented by sticking different-sized sponge to pieces of wood to give a good "handle" for the less able child. Try your own variations.

Applying the paint.   Getting the paint onto the potatoes or sponges may prove messy. Try putting the paint into a shallow tray such as the plastic trays meat is packed in when bought in a supermarket, or, even better, cut a piece of thin sponge to fit in the bottom of such a tray and soak it in the paint. This way there is little chance of spilling the paint.

Choosing the place.   Once the child understands what to do, this activity can be used like a game. Try taking it in turns to make a mark, and each time it is your turn, say where you are putting your mark; for example, "I am putting mine opposite your mark" or "I am putting this one beside yours." Or say "Guess where I am putting my next one?" In this way the child's awareness of place is heightened. It is possible to play this kind of game even with a child with no real language, so don't be afraid to try even if you are doing most of the talking.

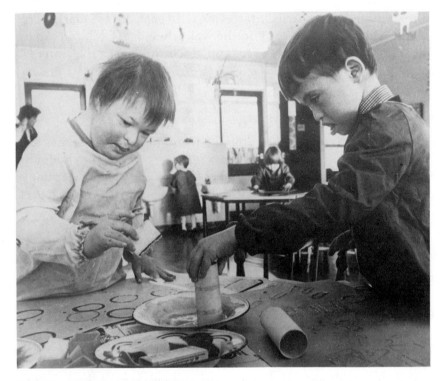

FIGURE 5.13. Making marks by printing.

PICTURE MAKING
WITH PASTA OR BUTTONS

Most grocery stores or supermarkets sell a variety of interestingly shaped pasta, and sometimes beans and peas of different colors. Pictures and designs can be made by arranging pasta or beans on a background and glueing them in place. Make a collection of different kinds of pasta or beans and store them in transparent jars. (You may find other uses for them as well, such as making rattles, threading them on string, or pressing them into clay.) The background for these pictures has to be fairly substantial, perhaps fairly thick cardboard. Begin using a board about the size of a magazine so that it is easy to see where the pieces are to be placed. Do not make the card so big that there is no space on the work surface for putting the loose pasta (see Figure 5.14).

The method of sticking is fairly complicated and many children will need help. The easiest way is to spread glue onto the board and place the pasta into the glue. A fairly able child will be able to learn

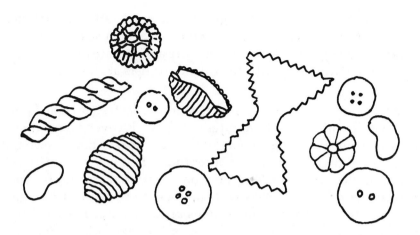

FIGURE 5.14. Buttons, beans, and pasta for making patterns.

how to do this, but the less able children will need help, so for these, paste the board ready for use.

It will be necessary to demonstrate the idea of the activity to your child: choosing a piece of pasta or a bean, picking it up, and placing it on the ready glued board. Say what you are doing, perhaps talking about the different kinds of shapes or colors you have to choose from. To begin with, use only a limited range either of beans or pasta, so that you can concentrate on the shape differences or the color. Encourage your child to talk about the pieces he or she chooses, so that the child becomes able to tell you the differences he or she sees. Again, don't be put off talking to your child if he or she cannot respond in the same way. The child can probably understand more than you think. Very often, conversations of a kind are possible even without words.

MAKING MARKS IN CLAY

Simply by prodding and poking clay with the fingers, many different marks can be made. Many more can be made by pressing objects into clay or scraping things along the clay.

Marks can be made on lumps of clay or on a flattened surface. At this stage you may find it easiest to encourage mark making on flat clay. It may be roughly flattened between the hands, or beaten on the table with the fist, or carefully rolled with a rolling pin. As it is quite difficult and hard work to flatten clay, don't be afraid to provide a ready flattened clay surface for your child to work on, but encourage those with the strength and interest to attempt to flatten a piece for themselves. (You might introduce the use of the rolling pin at a later stage, but feel that it is more appropriate for children to attempt to flatten clay with their hands or fists at this stage.)

Prodding and poking with the fingers.   Children will often prod and poke clay with their fingers in natural curiosity, discovering what clay feels like and the kinds of marks they can make. Encourage and extend this interest by finding other things that will make patterns in clay. Collect a few smallish common objects that are easy for your child to get hold of. Objects with an uneven or rough surface give the best patterns. Some suggestions are a fir cone, a piece of tree bark, a rough stone, a piece of string, or a dinner fork. Spend some time working with your child, trying out different ways of making marks, but also allow time for the children to explore on their own (see Figure 5.15).

Feeling the results.   As with comb painting (earlier in this chapter), the textured surface of clay is as much fun to feel as it is to look at. Allow any pieces of decorated clay to dry out and become hard. The texture can be felt more easily when the clay is dry because the handling won't smudge the surface. When clay is completely dried out, it can be baked or fired to make it more solid (see Appendix A). Clay does not have to be fired, but remember that dry, unbaked clay is very brittle and breaks easily. Try to arrange to bake some pieces; these can be handled most freely and be kept as a permanent reminder and record of work done.

FIGURE 5.15.   Things that will make marks in clay.

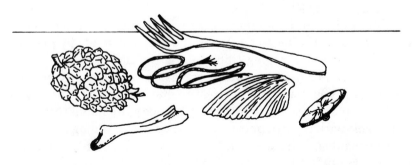

MATERIALS

The following list of materials looks long, but it is not intended to discourage you. It includes materials used for all the activities mentioned. Some materials will have to be bought and may not be very cheap, but I have tried to suggest materials that can be begged from neighbors and factories or saved from household rubbish as well. Once you have your eye tuned to what will be of use, I feel sure that your collection of useful bits and pieces will grow quickly. Certainly don't feel that it is necessary to get everything together before making a start.

PAINTING TOOLS AND MATERIALS

Paints.   Finger paints can be bought commercially, as specially prepared finger paints. It is also possible to mix a suitably thick paint by adding cold water paste or acrylic glue to poster colors. Remember to add extra water, particularly with cold water paste. Water-based poster colors are useful too. A limited number of colors is sufficient to begin with. Choose the primary colors (red, yellow, and blue) to start with, as other colors can be mixed from these if desired.

Ready-mix paints will become a useful addition, but may not be necessary yet. Ready-mix paints are good for squeezy painting. Each sort of paint has different qualities, and you may like to explore the use of others.

Brushes.   Choose large brushes, both flat and round, with plenty of firm bristles and a good handle. Small household paintbrushes can be useful as long as you have paint jars with big enough mouths for the brushes. A fat, short-bristled brush, such as a shaving brush, might be fun to experiment with. I have also experimented with a painting roller, but consider the space available before embarking upon this idea.

Sponges can be used instead of brushes, or made into "brushes" when tied to sticks. Cuts of foam rubber will do, or any ordinary household sponge that can be cut up to suit.

Things to draw with.   The main feature of the things you collect to draw with is that they be large, so that they are easy to grip and the mark made is a definite one and easy to see. Thick pencils, large wax crayons, and thick felt pens are good. The latter may be suitable only

51

toward the end of this stage, as too much pressure will soon ruin a felt pen.

Paper. Paper needs to be big and fairly strong. Colored construction paper is suitable, but can be expensive. Paper manufacturers or printers may have suitable wastepaper. I found a printer who threw away posters; the back of this paper is marvelous to work on. Another manufacturer gave away cuts of thin white cardboard.

Cold water or wallpaper paste. This is for mixing with powder colors for painting, finger painting, and comb painting. Store in an airtight container.

Acrylic glue or gesso. Use for mixing with paints to achieve thickness and texture.

Transparent or masking tape. This is useful for sticking paper to the table to keep it still, or hanging the finished picture on the wall.

Cardboard. Fairly thick cardboard, preferably quite substantial, is useful for making the combs and mounting pasta collage work.

Old squeezy dishwashing liquid bottles. These can be used either for storing paint that has been mixed or for trailing paint in squeezy paintings.

Jars and cans. These can be used both for the storage of paints and for putting paint into for use. Powder paint must be stored in airtight containers, either as powder or when mixed with water. Wide-based containers with large openings are most suitable for putting paint in; they are stable and make the dipping of brushes in and out easy. For those preferring them, nonspill paint cans can be bought.

Brown mailing tape. This is a must in the art room. It can be used at all stages and for many different things, but mainly for sticking sheets of paper together.

CLAY TOOLS AND MATERIALS
Clay and/or playdough (see Appendix A). Playdough can be made from equal quantities of flour and salt mixed with a small amount of

water. If put in an airtight bag or container, this can be stored in the refrigerator for quite a long time. Cake colors can be used to dye playdough. They are cheap and harmless.

Scraper.   Scrapers can be bought made from rubber or metal. Both can be used to smooth the surface of a piece of clay work, although this use is too sophisticated at this stage. The metal scraper is essential from the beginning to clean the table or boards after use. Using the flat edge of the scraper, flat surfaces can be easily scraped clean.

Cutting wire.   Cutting wires can be bought made up like a cheese cutter, a wooden handle on each end, or the wire can be bought separately and the wooden ends made from doweling. The wire will break quite easily, so it is a good idea to have some "loose" wire to make replacement cutters, whether you use your own or bought toggle ends.

Tools for using with clay.   There is no need for any actual tools at this stage. Collect objects that make interesting marks in clay, such as wire mesh, fir cones, combs, string, feathers, and so on. These can be collected with the help of your child over a period of time. The collection once begun will grow almost of its own accord!

A wooden board or canvas is necessary as a base on which to use the clay.

6

Activities for Stages 3 and 4

STAGE 3: MAKING THE SAME
MARK AGAIN

STAGE 4: MAKING SOMETHING
STAND FOR SOMETHING ELSE

As in Chapter 5, two closely linked development stages are discussed in this chapter. Because these are closely related stages, the activities suggested are suitable to both levels of development—more complex ideas developing from simpler beginnings.

   The activities in this chapter are designed to encourage children who have already acquired sufficient motor skills to repeat simple marks, and the perception to recognize them. During this stage there is likely to emerge an increasing balance between large extravagant movements and smaller ones. A child will probably become more aware of the edges of the paper when drawing and painting, and the circle or oval is likely to have particular importance.

   Children will probably now begin to name the objects they have made or drawn. To start, a child may give a name to shapes and patterns, but these images will not be instantly (if at all) recognizable; they will not look like the names given them, although the same kind of pattern or shape may repeatedly be given the same name. This is natural, and gradually the images made will become more recognizable; that is, they will look more like the name given them.

Children will probably be able to learn a number of new skills during this stage. The activities involve using a rolling pin, glue, or scissors.

GENERAL HINTS

TALKING ABOUT WHAT HAPPENS
All practical activities involve learning based on action; learning that can only be acquired through doing. A child can learn to scribble only by picking up a pencil and making the movements; he or she can get better at drawing only by practicing making the marks. But it is sometimes possible to help this kind of learning by pointing out to a child what he or she has done and what has happened as a result. So, sometimes spend time talking with your child about an activity and about what he or she has done, pointing out his or her achievements.

NAMING PICTURES
It is quite usual for children to begin naming the marks they make at this stage; even marks that don't look like anything in particular to us may be given names. If your child is happy to talk about his or her work, it can be a ready source of conversation. Your comments should be confirming. Reinforce this early naming process, even if it appears to make little sense, as it makes good sense to the child and to his or her development. Although a child may begin to name the marks he or she makes and thus make connections between things and the work, be wary of making connections on behalf of a child. It may be helpful to say a mark that your child has made reminds you of something, or that it is like something, but don't tell the child what he or she has drawn, as you will probably be wrong. Your comments can encourage a child to notice more about an object named when he or she looks at it again, and you may sometimes help by asking what your child has drawn. But don't insist that your child tell you about the pictures. Simply be a receptive audience if the child wants to talk.

REMEMBERING
A child's power of recall begins to grow at this stage, and it becomes possible to link things that are made or drawn with other things that are not visible at the moment of speaking. A child can

begin to make the connection between a photograph of something and the memory of the real thing, so it can be fun to take photographs of outings or holidays and have them available during art activities.

LIMIT THE POSSIBILITIES

It remains important not to confuse your child by offering too many alternatives at any one time. Particularly when introducing a new idea, it is sensible to limit the possibilities of choice to one or two. But as children develop, they will be less easily overwhelmed and may benefit from access to a greater variety of tools and materials than previously. If equipment is easily available, children may find their own ways of developing or extending a suggested idea, perhaps combining two ideas or methods in a way their teacher had not thought of.

To find a happy balance between limited choice and free access to materials may be difficult. Materials and tools used regularly by your child should be always kept in the same place and in easy reach of your child. Encourage him or her to help in the getting out and putting away of the materials so that the child becomes familiar with the organization of activities and learns where the materials are kept. Should the occasion arise that your child wants more or additional equipment, he or she should be able to find them quite easily, but not be confused by their presence.

LEARNING TO USE SIMPLE TOOLS

It is impossible to predict how physical development will correlate with development of perceptions. Some children may be ready to tackle the use of simple tools, such as a pottery cutting knife or a pair of scissors, very early in their general development; others may have difficulties for much longer. Try to judge by the ease with which the child does other things, his or her readiness to try these new activities. Watch your child's approach to other tasks that require the use of simple tools. Observe, for instance, the way the child uses a knife and fork, or how well he or she controls a toothbrush. Attempt to introduce these new activities when your child seems ready and willing to try them.

IT ALL TAKES TIME

All new learning takes time, and it is often necessary to repeat something several times before really understanding how to do it. In this stage, use a rolling pin and scissors. When introducing these or other new activities, do not be disappointed if you seem to have no success at first. It takes time to understand the movements necessary to perform these skills and to learn how to control them. Introduce new activities step by step, doing a little more each time. Never expect more than partial mastery of something. Be sensitive to and appreciative of success, and show your pleasure. Not only does this help your child, but in recognizing success you will feel encouraged yourself.

THINGS TO DO

Getting It Better

We all know the saying "practice makes perfect," and there is no doubt about its wisdom. Practicing something does help us to get better at it.

The activities described in this chapter are intended to encourage the practice of skills already discovered; they will be extensions of activities already described. The suggestions are designed to reinforce learning that began in previous explorations in drawing, painting, and clay work.

The next few ideas are designed to help a child to get better control of actions and to encourage the ability to recognize shapes and patterns.

FINDING AN ORDER

As a natural extension of the previous random scribbling (see Chapter 5), children will begin to make some more controlled movements while drawing. It is likely that children will make circular movements on paper, so that circles or ovals will appear spontaneously in the scribble. Gradually, these shapes will become more refined and children will begin to draw them by themselves.

Continue to encourage your child to draw freely for pleasure. Gradually, as circle or oval shapes appear, scribbling will take on less importance. Finally, the shapes will be drawn on their own and appear as little pictures instead of in the middle of a scribble (see Figure 6.1). When these shapes begin to appear, even as part of a scribble, draw attention to them, show interest in them, praise them. When you draw the child's attention to them in this way, your

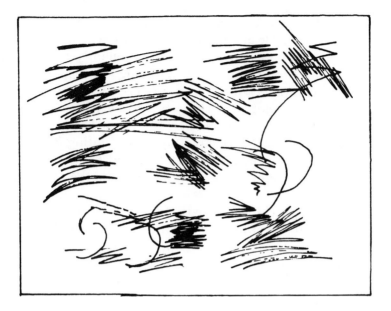

FIGURE 6.1. Finding an order: Circles discovered in a scribble.

child will be encouraged to look at them more closely and may be encouraged to find a way of repeating similar marks again.

The development from scribbling to drawing isolated marks is a natural one that can be aided by drawing attention to it when it begins to happen spontaneously. Try hanging pictures on the wall at this stage to give your child plenty of opportunity to look again and see for him- or herself the order of patterns and shapes the child has made.

MAKING THE SAME ORDER AGAIN

Give plenty of opportunities for your child to make marks in all sorts of different materials. As well as using drawing materials such as pens, crayons, and felt pens, offer paints as an alternative "drawing" medium. The flowing quality of paint gives it a special importance to some children, but can prove difficult for others to handle. Be sensitive to these difficulties and make things as easy as possible for your child. One particular difficulty with painting is the need to keep dipping a paintbrush into paint to keep it damp enough to flow over the paper. Always provide large brushes at this stage, as they hold the most paint. To help keep the paints and brushes clean, provide one brush for each color provided. This eliminates the need to rinse the brushes each time a new color is used. Special nonspill paint cans are available and preferred in many schools. These cans have tops that not only prevent paint from spilling out readily, but also provide space for only one brush, leaving little opportunity for mistakes. Unfortunately, with these cans it is usually impossible for a child to tell what color he or she is about to use because the cans and lids are opaque. If you choose to use nonspill cans, label them with colored paper as described in Squeezy Painting (Chapter 5). Large-based cans for paint are impractical in most households, but if the base is large enough, the cans are stable and the colors can be seen.

Free painting is closely related to free drawing and gives similar opportunity for discovering special marks. Watch to see if your child makes similar marks in his or her drawing and painting. If so, point them out so that the child can appreciate them too. Try hanging two pictures, a drawing and a painting, showing similarities, beside one another so that your child has opportunities to make the connections.

I SPY

As well as simply pointing out the similarity between marks that a child has repeated in several pictures, try playing a game such as "I spy," where you choose a particular mark and help your child to discover it in his or her own work. This can be successfully played using colors as well as marks. Try saying something like "I can see a round mark in your picture." Point out the circle, perhaps drawing it with your finger. Get your child to repeat the same action, pointing out the circle, drawing it with his or her finger. Encourage the child to say he or she can see a round mark.

COPY CAT

Try also a copying game. Choose from your child's picture a mark repeated fairly often. Make a drawing of this mark yourself on a separate sheet of paper and encourage your child to copy you! In this game your child is only repeating, again, a mark he or she has already made spontaneously several times before. You have not really invented new skills for your child at all, simply reinforced old ones. By drawing attention to certain marks in this way, you can help a child to explore and remember how to control spontaneous movements to produce more deliberate marks.

DRAWING IN
SLIP—SLIP TRAILING

Slip trailing is a well-known method of decorating flat or almost flat clay surfaces. It is similar in many ways to the painting technique described in Chapter 5, where paint was squeezed from liquid bottles. For slip trailing, flat clay is used as a base instead of paper and clay slip instead of paint. As slip flows very easily from a trailer, the amount of pressure used must be carefully controlled, so this is a good activity for children practicing to control their movements.

Although slip trailing is usually only part of a lengthier process, treat it also as an end in itself, encouraging your child to watch the results of squeezing and moving (see Figure 6.2).

Roll a piece of clay out flat and use it as a base to make a pattern.

FIGURE 6.2. Using a slip trailer.

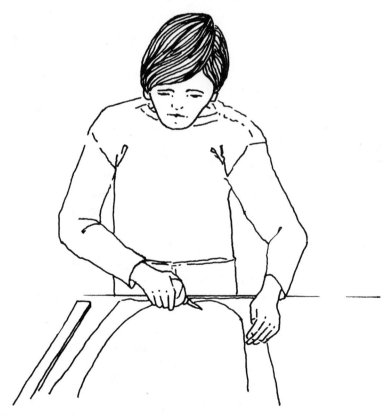

Mix slip as described in Appendix A and color with oxides as desired. Use only two or three colors. Successful results can be achieved by using simple earthy colors.

Fill the slip trailers by squeezing the rubber bulbs to get rid of all the air, then put the nozzle into the slip and gradually release the bulb. The trailer will suck up the slip as the bulb regains its shape.

Simple but interesting patterns can be made by experimenting with different movements and the amount of pressure used, so slip trailing can offer yet another opportunity for children to practice more controlled mark making.

DRAWING IN CLAY

There are two ways in which clay can be a medium for drawing. Simple pictures can be scratched into flattened clay, or clay "worms" can be placed on a background and used as lines to make up a drawing.

Scratching into clay.   Making pictures in flattened clay is similar, in many ways, to making the textural patterns suggested in Chapter 5, but with a new-found order imposed on them. Clay rolled flat with a rolling pin is most suitable for making drawings with sharpened sticks, skewers, or a wooden pottery knife, but clay roughly flattened with the fist or palm makes a reasonable base for drawing, too. Show your child how a line can be made by moving a fairly thin and pointed tool across the clay, just as marks were made by pressing various objects into the clay before. Provide alternative tools for your child to experiment with, perhaps even a blunt pencil or ballpoint pen. Look out for similarities (and differences) between clay pictures and ordinary drawings. Share with your child the similarities you find.

Drawing with clay worms.   Children who have learned how to roll clay worms under their hands (see Figure 5.6, Chapter 5) have another way of making drawings. By placing clay worms on a board or clay base, turning, joining, and breaking them as required, they can use the worms as lines, just as they do drawn lines, to create pictures. Show your child how a "picture" can be made in this way by making a simple pattern or picture yourself. Or simply encourage the laying on and pressing down of clay worms without worrying about what the result looks like. Your child will invent his or her own patterns or pictures once he or she understands how to use the clay worms.

Combining textures, marks, and worm lines.   There is no reason for keeping the two ways of drawing in clay separate. Encourage your child to experiment by making marks in the clay with his or her fingers, with a drawing tool, by pressing textured objects into the clay, and by laying on clay worms (see Figure 6.3). Try also flattening the clay worms with a rolling pin.

So as not to overwhelm your child, or make the experiment too difficult, introduce this combination of ideas only when the alternative methods are familiar. Some children are naturally more likely to experiment than others, and for them it may be enough to introduce the alternative forms. But for many it will be necessary to suggest combining two or more methods and to provide the necessary tools. Talk to your child about what he or she is doing and involve the child in deliberately making simple choices.

PUSHING AND PULLING CLAY
INTO SHAPE
While exploring clay, children will have been squashing, squeezing, and rolling it into different kinds of shapes. Each child

FIGURE 6.3. Drawing with clay worms and by scratching on clay.

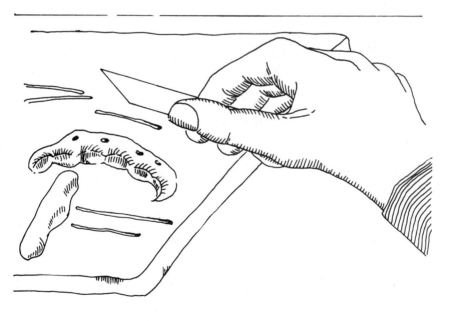

will have made his or her own discoveries and can be helped to invent even more new ways of making shapes (see Figure 5.5, Chapter 5). Continue to share with your child the excitement of handling clay and making shapes. Encourage the child to make those he or she finds easiest and try to help find ways of extending these into new shapes. Rather than showing your child how to make completely new shapes, find ways to demonstrate how shapes he or she has already made can be altered by pinching or squashing them in different ways, by flattening them or joining them together.

Making objects in clay.   All sorts of objects, even animals or people, can be made by squashing, squeezing, or pulling clay from an original ball, or by pushing several small pieces together to form a more complex shape. Remember that it is unlikely that a child will be able to make a recognizable object, but encourage your child to experiment forming shapes in clay. Not only does this encourage physical dexterity, but it also serves an important role in the child's growing ability to imagine things. Do not be upset if your child gives a name to very crude forms, or even to a ball of clay. Accept the name, enjoy the object, and later try to find means of introducing new ways of handling the clay, ways that will eventually help your child to modify the crude images to be more like the name he or she has given them.

THE BEGINNING
OF BUILDING POTS

Pots are containers made especially for keeping things in, and clay is the traditional material from which they are made. There is no reason for your child to make pots, but it is noticeable that many children choose to make cups, saucers, or plates among their first creations. These are all fairly simple objects with which children are familiar. Simple pots such as these can be made in the hands without the use of tools, and children often invent their own ways of making them without help.

Here are two simple methods you might demonstrate to your child as alternative ways of using clay, but without insisting he or she make a shape exactly like your own.

Show your child how a hole can be made in a ball of clay by pushing a finger or thumb into it. Depending on the size of the ball of clay, the sides can be pressed and molded to make different shapes.

Alternatively, simple flat-bottomed pots can be made from flattened clay by pulling the edges up to stand upright to form the sides.

Both these methods may be used by your child to make a variety of different objects.

Stretching Out

All the suggestions in Reaching Out (Chapter 5) can be used by children working at this stage, too.

FLOOR AND WALL PAINTING

Many children will need reminding to stretch out and reach as far as they can, so continue to offer your child the alternatives of painting on the floor or on paper on a wall or at an easel (see Figures 6.4 and 6.5). Offer your child paper of different sizes, sometimes a very large sheet, and encourage him or her to be aware of the possibilities offered because of size variation. Help your child to understand that his or her pictures have to be small to fit on a small piece of paper, but that there is a choice when given a larger sheet.

ROLLING OUT CLAY

Rolling clay requires a different kind of stretching out, and the amount of clay to be rolled out determines the need for stretching. Rolling clay also requires physical control and strength. This is not a difficult skill to learn, for it uses similar skills to rolling clay worms or snakes under one's hand, but it does require much more pressure and encourages a child to stretch out and reach farther.

The flat clay produced will have many uses, some described in this chapter and others described in more advanced stages. Its simplest use is as a new base for making texture marks and pictures.

Rolling out with a rolling pin is best done standing up (see Figure 6.6). Begin by demonstrating how to do it. Try standing behind your child, one arm each side of him or her, and make your child go through the action with you. Make your child put his or her hands on top of yours to feel the action, and then try with yours on top. To "get it right" needs practice and patience, but once the idea is established the skill is quickly learned. Many children have difficulty putting enough pressure on the rolling pin and need assistance for some time. To help your child to get it right, take it in turns to do some rolling each, or reward a good effort by finishing the job. For

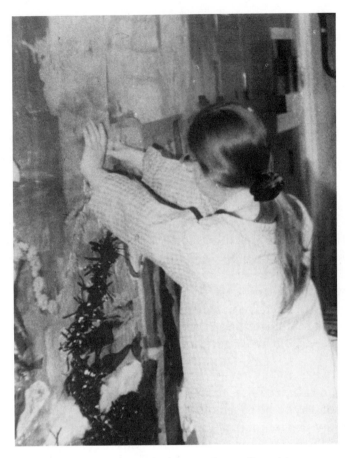

FIGURE 6.4. Stretching up—working on a large collage picture.

children having considerable difficulties, practice with playdough (or even real pastry), which is much softer.

Clay is best rolled out on a piece of canvas, and if an even thickness is required, place the clay between two battens (strips of wood) and rest the ends of the rolling pin on them. Thus the clay can be rolled only as thin as the thickness of the battens and will be the same thickness all over.

Finding the Difference

As a child's awareness of things becomes better, he or she will gain pleasure in handling, sorting, and using a greater variety of materials.

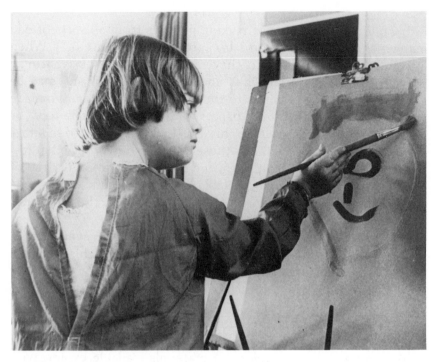

FIGURE 6.5. Painting at an easel.

FIGURE 6.6. Rolling out clay
with a rolling pin.

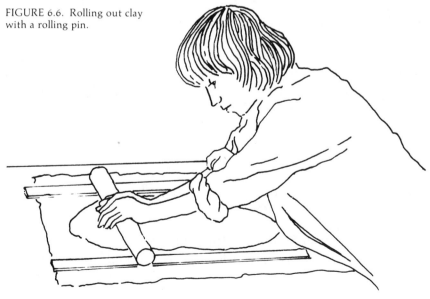

COLLAGE

Collage is a method of making pictures from all sorts of odd materials, fixed together on a background (see Figure 6.7). When introducing a collage activity, have an open mind as to what may prove interesting to your child and as to how he or she may be encouraged to attach things to the picture. Pictures can be made from such things as colored papers, photographs, bottle tops, or wood shavings; you can add to this list. It may be useful to separate materials into different kinds—those that are shiny, those that feel soft, and so on. To begin with, limit the number or variety of different materials that are available so that your child is not overwhelmed by the choices. Help your child to notice the difference between things by offering contrasting materials.

Pictures can be put together with glue, staples, or even stitches (see suggestions under Making a Scrapbook later in this chapter). This kind of activity can be enjoyable and useful in itself. A number of skills are being exercised, including those of selecting and arranging, tearing or cutting, sticking, stapling, or sewing. The pictures made may not represent anything, or even appear to be organized at all; they may be just a pleasurable collection of bits and pieces. But encourage your child to explore the materials available, explore with him or her, and talk about the quality of the materials. For example, share the fact that a bottle top is shiny, or that wood shavings are curved. It may be useful to comment that the materials are like something else. But refrain from saying that part of the picture represents something else; leave this to the child.

Collage work can also be linked to drawing and painting activities. For example, a child able to draw only a kind of "matchstick" man with bulbous head will be able to recognize photographs of people and may enjoy sticking them beside his or her own drawings, or even drawing on top of them.

FEELING THE DIFFERENCE—
FABRIC COLLAGE

For children who have mastered the use of scissors, making fabric collages can be an extension to the collage pictures described earlier. They will also be exercising selection of materials, according to how they feel.

Have available fabrics of different textures. For those unable to use scissors, cut fabrics into fairly small pieces of different shapes, so that they are ready to stick on a background piece of paper or

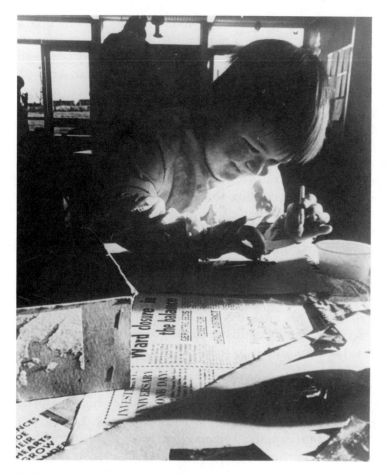

FIGURE 6.7. Selecting and pasting down.

cardboard. Among your collection, have fabrics that are soft, such as fur or velvet, some that are harsh, such as canvas, others that are ridged like cord, and so on. Make the collection as varied and as interesting to feel as possible.

Attempt to involve your child in an exploration of the differences in the feel between the fabrics, share in this experience, and talk about the textures you can feel.

PAPER TEARING

Paper can be divided into smaller pieces by tearing or by cutting. To understand that paper can be divided up is important to the idea of cutting paper, and so paper tearing can be a preliminary skill to paper cutting. But it is also a valuable activity in its own right. Although cutting may be a more difficult skill, and cutting shapes more precise, this does not make it *better*. The quality of the edge of the torn paper is different and more interesting than a cut edge. A torn piece of paper has a wavy or jagged edge, a cut piece has a straight, hard edge.

It is extremely difficult to tear paper with skill and control. The physical skills used are varied and complex, so try to find a way that suits your child best. Small shapes can be torn from paper if the paper is turned around—rough strips can be simply pulled and torn, or be controlled by moving the fingers along the strip as it tears. Encourage the use of torn paper in collage, for weaving or sticking paper shapes on to a background. The latter provides a record of achievement and opportunities for selection and choice in placing the shapes made.

The qualities of torn and cut paper are very different—should the precise shape of the paper pieces become of greater interest to your child than the quality of the torn edge, begin to encourage the use of scissors. The straight cut edge of paper produces clear shapes, whereas the edges made by tearing have more interesting qualities.

SIMPLE WEAVING

Weaving encourages the exploration and choice of materials, according to their color and texture. It is related to collage pictures, but requires fairly nimble fingers. Instead of choosing materials to stick onto a background sheet, choose threads and strips of paper or fabric to weave into one another. Weaving can be done very freely, without precision about alternate under-and-over threading.

Weaving requires some kind of frame, either one especially made or an old picture frame. Put an equal number of tacks along two opposite sides of the frame (we will call these two sides top and bottom) at about 1 cm (about 1/2 in.) intervals. These tacks will support the first threads, which will, in turn, form the basis for the weaving. Wind wool or string up and down the frame, taking it around two tacks at the top, then two at the bottom, and so on (see Figure 6.8). When all the tacks have been used, tie off the thread securely. Other threads, material strips, or even feathers or colored paper can now be threaded in and out across the first threads to make the finished fabric (see Figure 6.9).

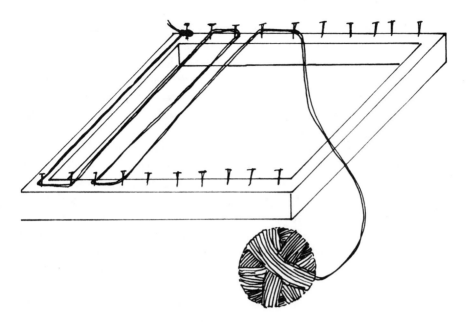

FIGURE 6.8. Threading a weaving frame.

FIGURE 6.9. The sort of pattern made by weaving.

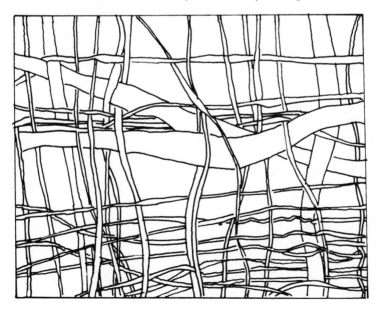

Most children will probably enjoy threading bits and pieces in and out with their fingers, but a cardboard "needle" can be used. A cardboard needle is a strip of stiff cardboard, cut slightly longer than the width of the frame. It has a fairly large hole in one end. To use it, weave the cardboard in and out of the threads on the frame, thread whatever fabric or twine is to be used through the eye of the needle, then pull the needle through.

Encourage your child to explore the possible materials and to use whatever takes his or her fancy. Silver paper and cellophane both produce fascinating effects in among more ordinary fibers, such as wool. Don't plan to have a weaving finished at one sitting; it is work to go back to several times. The finished piece can be lifted off the tacks fairly easily and mounted between two cardboard frames. Depending on the sort of materials used, it may be fun to display weaving on a window, so that light can shine through, showing up the textural, semitransparent quality of the work. The discovery of these qualities may provide your child with an idea for another piece of work, making particular use of transparent materials.

SEE-THROUGH PICTURES

Much of the pleasure in work at all stages, but in particular at this stage, has to do with the quality of materials and marks made. Experimentation with different kinds of materials remains important. See-through pictures have a special, almost magical, quality, as they change according to the amount of light shining through them.

Cellophane and tissue paper are the most common transparent materials, and these can be used in weaving, or can be stuck, overlapping one another, across a paper or cardboard frame to produce an effect similar to that of a stained glass window.

To make a frame, choose a piece of paper or thin cardboard of the size required for the finished work. Around the edge draw a frame about 20 cm (nearly 8 in.) wide. Using scissors or a knife, cut out the center, leaving the frame ready for use. Strips or shapes of transparent materials can be placed across the frame and glued at both ends onto the edges.

Encourage your child to discover what happens when two or more pieces of tissue or cellophane overlap. Don't worry about what the picture looks like, but enjoy the effects of making colors for the light to shine through. If the finished work is put on a window, look for where the colors are projectd by the sun onto the floor or onto a wall inside the room.

Having Something to Talk About

It has probably become noticeable that your child has now increased powers of recall, that he or she can more and more recognize things from previous occasions or other places.

MAKING A SCRAPBOOK

Making a scrapbook relies on two difficult skills—those of glueing and of cutting with scissors. Learning to glue correctly requires close supervision in the early stages, as your child will need reminding to put the glue onto the back of the picture he or she has chosen, and then to turn it over to stick it in place. Almost inevitably a child will begin by putting the glue on the face of the picture he or she wants to stick. While helping children who are learning this skill, remind them constantly what they have to do, telling them as well as showing them the successful way.

Using scissors requires complex skills, for they need to be opened and closed by the control of one hand, as well as to be steered in the desired direction. Beginners' scissors can be purchased, and these are a help because they are designed so that pressure is required only to close them; they spring open again automatically, ready for the next cut.

Making a scrapbook is not an easy exercise, but one particularly useful for children whose physical and perceptual skills are developing well, but who are reluctant to use messier materials. Scrapbooks can be made from sheets of almost any large pieces of paper; brown wrapping paper is fine. Cut the sheets twice the size of a single page; fold them in half and either stitch or staple them together down the center fold to form a book. A special cover can be made from heavier paper or cardboard. It is difficult to recommend a size, but you probably should not make one smaller than about 39 x 25 cm (about 15 x 10 in.).

The scraps used to stick into the book can be anything that attracts or interests your child. Save old magazines, cards, and calendars; they are a good source of a variety of pictures. One most effective scrapbook contained the Sunday news supplement and television guide introductions to television programs recognized by a young man I taught. He also collected photographs of well-known personalities. Attempt to provide for an individual's interest, rather than insist that he or she be interested in what is available.

It may sometimes be useful to begin a scrapbook with a child *before* he or she has acquired all the necessary skills. The choosing of the entries can be done by the child, but you will do some of the work, perhaps the cutting and helping with the glueing. With encouragement, this kind of introduction may lead the child gradually to do more alone, until he or she is able to take over from you.

DO YOU KNOW WHAT THIS IS?

This art room "game" is good in odd minutes, or for longer periods. Make a simple line drawing of an everyday object. Ask your child (or group of children) how soon he or she can recognize what you are drawing, as you are drawing it. Allow the children to play the drawing role as well, if they will, and you do the guessing. Although it is very unlikely that they will be able to draw a recognizable picture themselves, the attempt will be good practice. Keep the game very light; play it just for fun.

MATERIALS

There is never any need to get rid of materials acquired for activities described in an earlier section; those suggested in Chapter 5 form the basis of a collection that can be added to at any point. Included in the list below are those materials already mentioned, with comments only on new materials and new uses for old materials.

PAINTING AND
OTHER MATERIALS

Paints.   Ready-mixed acrylics and/or poster paints can be useful additions at any stage, but particularly if your child gets obvious pleasure from painting. Both ready-mix paint, which has a polyvinyl acrylic base, and poster paints, which are water based, give good strong colors. Special care is needed in storing and dispensing poster and acrylic paints so that they are not wasted or spoiled by drying out or being made dirty with unwashed brushes. Brushes used in acrylic paints should be washed thoroughly after use. Add to the basic color selection to give more variety and possible choices. Suggested colors to add are black, white, green, orange, and purple.

Brushes.   Add some smaller brushes to your collection. They should still have long handles with firm bristles and can be round or flat. Sponges still have many uses as substitute brushes.

Drawing materials.   Pencils may be used for drawing more frequently at this stage; and add some slightly thinner ones. Finer wax crayons may be useful, but will break easily if subjected to too much pressure. Colored pencil crayons may be useful, but again the points will break easily if used with too much pressure. Use discretion here, for it is no use attempting to use materials that are obviously too delicate for your child. Stick to the large robust pencils and crayons until your child's control is sufficiently good to make them a worthwhile investment.

Ballpoint pens could be tried, and finer felt-tipped pens too.

Wax pastels, although expensive and rather quickly used up, do produce particularly beautiful colors, and might be an occasional treat.

Paper.   Any large paper you have acquired will still be useful, and colored construction paper is ideal, but it may be possible to use some smaller and thinner paper than before. A great deal depends on individual development and the control of pressure. Have some colored paper available if possible; sometimes offer your child a choice. Even the simple process of choosing a sheet of paper is important.

Adhesives.   Cold water paste is good for sticking paper as well as for mixing with paints. Acrylic glue will be particularly useful for making collages with cloth. Also use contact and other sticky paper.

Collage materials.   Begin a collection of colored papers. Christmas wrapping paper or colored paper, bags, buttons, ribbons, sequins, and so on; the list could be endless. Keep a cardboard box in which to store things that you come across and find interesting.

Scissors.   Some children will be ready to use scissors at this stage. It may be helpful to get a pair of beginner's scissors that open with a gentle spring, thus needing only a firm grip and pressure to close them to cut (see Figure 6.10).

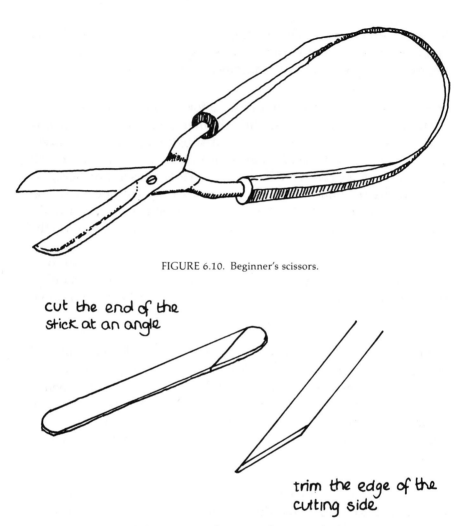

FIGURE 6.10. Beginner's scissors.

cut the end of the
stick at an angle

trim the edge of the
cutting side

FIGURE 6.11. Making a wooden pottery knife.

Old frames.   Old picture frames are useful as frames for weaving. Tacks are then pushed into the frames along two opposite sides at approximately 1 cm (nearly ½ in.) intervals.

MATERIALS FOR USE WITH CLAY
A wooden knife for scratching, marking, and cutting clay can be made from a wooden popsicle stick (see Figure 6.11), or bought commercially.

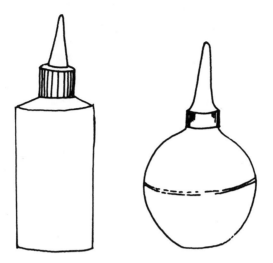

FIGURE 6.12. Slip trailers.

ADDITIONAL TOOLS
The following additional tools may be useful:

Scraper.

Cutting wire.

Brush for use with slip or water.

Airtight container in which to store a small quantity of made-up slip.

Rolling pin (an ordinary wooden rolling pin will do, and a perfectly plain one is best).

Wooden battens—two pieces of wood about 40 cm (nearly 16 in.) long, 3 cm (about 1 in.) by 0.5 cm (¼ in.) thick. These are used when rolling clay to an even thickness.

Slip trailers. These must be bought commercially and are designed especially for the job (see Figure 6.12).

7

Activities for Stage 5

STAGE 5: REMEMBERING THE PAST

Activities at stage 5 are designed for children who have sufficient control of their movements to draw or make something requiring a lot of skill. Although the images that they make may still seem odd or distorted, they are often quite recognizable as something. Even the least clear images are likely to have an individual order about them and to be made with purpose and control.

Suggestions at this stage are intended to encourage greater control of actions. It is suggested that both scissors and simple wooden pottery knives be used. A child's increased ability to remember things is encouraged, and activities for which a number of small steps must be completed in the correct order are included. Children should be encouraged to look more closely at things about them and to share their experiences. Some group work at this stage may have particular advantages.

GENERAL HINTS

THE USE OF TOOLS
Your child's confidence to use simple tools should gradually have been growing. Most children will be able to use, or be able to

learn to use, a wooden pottery knife for cutting clay, or scissors for cutting paper. For those having particular difficulties with either skill, find ways to help them learn a little at a time. A pottery knife can be used to chop clay worms in half, or for stabbing into clay to make texture patterns. Scissors can be used to divide paper strips into small pieces for collage or weaving. These examples hardly need the use of knife or scissors at all, but they give your child a little practice in handling and using the tools. Success at such simple tasks will help children to be more confident in trying more and different things.

BALANCE BETWEEN LEARNING NEW SKILLS AND EXPERIMENTING WITH OLD IDEAS

Especially when working with clay, it may be difficult to keep a balance between introducing new ideas and leaving time for exploration. It is important that children have plenty of time to work freely, finding their own ways of using materials, perhaps inventing their own modifications of learned skills.

Watch for signs that indicate that your child is ready to learn something new. He or she may simply ask to know how something is done, attempt to copy someone working at a more advanced stage, or seem bored with his or her own work.

Remember that children working in a group will learn from each other and often modify what they see to suit their own needs. Children will also copy adults, so continue to join in and help your child to learn.

THE USE OF MEMORY

Increasingly, a child will be able to remember things from the past. The child will be able to remember and recall things that have happened to him or her, and also ways of working and methods of doing things.

At this stage much drawing and painting can be based on things that have happened. Shared experiences outside the art room can be important. Photographs and mementoes can serve as reminders and prompt a child's memory.

Other activities suggested in this chapter, particularly those using clay, rely upon a child's remembering several simple steps that contribute toward one activity. Continue to encourage your child to organize the materials and equipment needed for an activity. Finding the things he or she needs and putting them away again is good training for more complex organization.

GROUP ACTIVITIES

At this stage children should sometimes be encouraged to work together to make a shared piece of work. Group work requires a number of children to cooperate with one another, to articulate and share their ideas, to share materials and space. To be successful, such an activity requires preparation and forethought.

Involve the children in the idea of making a picture together from the beginning. Help them to articulate ideas and to gather information as well as to organize their materials and equipment.

MAKING IT LOOK RIGHT

Much of the work done at this stage will be based on places, people, and things that the children know about. Most of the images will be fairly easy to recognize, but will not look exactly as you might expect them to. Certain distortions that it may be tempting to dismiss as inaccuracies will appear in the work. Some things you consider important will be missed completely. These distortions are better viewed as emphasis. Every emphasis will be on the things that these children find most important or enjoyable. Artists do this in their pictures, just as ordinary people do in recounting an experience. Be aware of the emphasis your child puts into artwork and learn from his or her pictures what the child finds most interesting and important.

THE USE OF MATERIALS

Continue to encourage your child to use a variety of art materials to make pictures for pleasure. Give access to paints, crayons, felt pens, wax crayons, pencils, and collage materials as before. If it is possible to keep materials where your child can see them and choose for him- or herself, all to the good. As art activities become increasingly self-motivated, your child will want to make his or her own choices. Try to provide a variety of paper of different sizes and colors.

Remember that many of the activities suggested in Chapter 6 will be continued into this stage, and that the methods and techniques learned will be used more confidently with greater practice.

THINGS TO DO

Awareness and Control of Self

This activity begins as a kind of awareness exercise, but it uses quite complex drawing skills. Children are also required to look at and compare similar shapes.

AM I AS BIG AS THAT?
HANDS AND FEET
In Chapter 5, "reaching out" activities were suggested to encourage your child to make hand prints on paper. Now try a comparison game by drawing around either hands or feet. Compare the size and shape of your child's hands with your own. It is easier to draw around someone else's hands and feet than your own, and feet are on the whole easier than hands. Show your child how to move the pencil around the foot, while keeping to the outline.

Make a pattern from the drawings. Having made the drawings, try some of the following ideas. Many patterns can be created using the shapes made by drawing around the hands or feet. Try drawing different hand shapes overlapping one another. The resulting line drawing could be painted or colored in. More complex line patterns can be made by using pens or crayons of different colors when drawing around the hands or feet. Try drawing the shapes on different colored papers, then cutting out and arranging various patterns. Finally, experiment by drawing around another object that your child is interested in. Try your own variations and experiments.

AM I AS LARGE AS THAT?
HEAD TO TOE
Although a child's awareness of things around him or her will be gradually improving, images of things and of him- or herself and work will continue to appear distorted. This distortion should be viewed as emphasis and has a particular value. But awareness of oneself, one's size, shape, and capabilities has special importance. To encourage this kind of awareness, make a life-size "portrait." This activity can be shared between two or more children, and it is best done with at least two. Children will be able to compare their size and shape and later their coloring. The activity needs lots of floor

space and a large wall space. A mirror must be available, ideally a full-length mirror such as a dressmaker's or wardrobe mirror.

Stick several pieces of paper together until you have made a piece at least as tall and as wide as your child. Stick the pieces together using masking tape, stuck on the wrong side. Encourage your child to help, holding the paper still or smoothing the tape; tell your child clearly what you want him or her to do, or show the child. Although the task will take longer than it would on your own, the extra time spent will be worthwhile.

One child has to lie down on the paper with arms beside his or her body. The second child then draws around the body. Of course, this is not as simple as it sounds, as bodies are not flat, and it is very easy, for instance, to push a pencil too far underneath the curve of the limbs, and so make a drawing of a very thin-looking person. Without actually doing it, guide the child making the drawing to hold the pencil as upright as possible, enabling him or her to get a fair likeness of the real shape of the model. Feet will always prove to be very difficult, and you will have to help out here, and do *your* best at finishing the feet.

Once the outline is complete, the "model" can get up and see the shape that has been drawn. This is a marvelously exciting time and observations can begin right away. Often children don't believe that they are "as big as that," but they can quickly and easily compare the size of their hands with those in the picture and perhaps with those of their friend.

To continue working on the picture, hang it on a wall so that the drawn figure confronts the real figure (see Figure 7.1). With the aid of a full-length mirror, enter into a comparing and matching game. First, "finish off" the drawing with details of clothing, facial features, hair, and so on. Continue the game to include color. Paint the figure as it really is. Children can be persuaded to wear the same clothes for more than one art lesson, or be encouraged to remember what they had on yesterday, or last week, when they last worked on the painting.

Adult help is essential to this work, for not only must the children be helped through conversation to compare themselves with their picture, but some of the necessary color mixing and matching will need adult help. Don't do the jobs for the children, but always encourage them to discover what must be done, with your help.

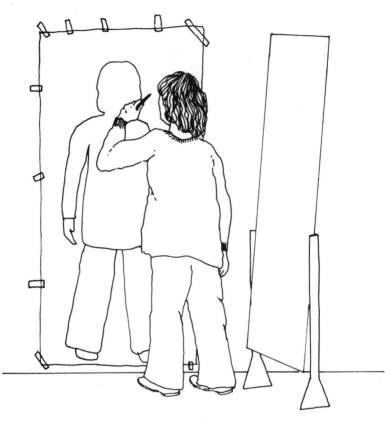

FIGURE 7.1. A head-to-toe portrait.

Getting the Right Things
in the Right Order

From the earliest experimental stage, children have been encouraged to make patterns in clay by pressing things into it. With their increased skills, children can progress to more detailed tasks.

MAKING AND DECORATING TILES

Making simple textured tiles is a good project for children at this stage. It is a familiar activity, altered to make use of new skills.

Many children working at this stage develop a strong sense of order, and love making repetitive patterns. Order, even of this simple kind, is worth encouraging, and tile making can give an alternative to drawing and painting. Encourage your child to use his or her strength to flatten the clay, either using the pressure of the palms of the hands, or with a rolling pin. Clay roughly flattened by hand will produce unpredictable shapes, whereas clay flattened with a rolling pin can be used for making several tiles all the same size.

Making several tiles the same size and shape.   To make tiles the same size, you have to cut around a template. A template is a shape or pattern, similar to a dressmaker's pattern, which is used as a guide to cut around. For clay work, it can be made from either paper or cardboard. You will probably have to help to make the template for this work, and a simple one suitable for use several times can be cut from a piece of fairly strong cardboard. The cardboard from the back of a writing pad will do, but cardboard with a shiny or very smooth surface would be even better, as this will absorb less moisture from the clay and, therefore, last longer. A square template about 10 x 10 cm (4 x 4 in.) is reasonably easy to handle in the beginning. All the rest of the work can be done by your child, with your help and guidance.

A ball of prepared clay should be rolled out, preferably on canvas. Use the wooden battens as a guide to correct and even thickness. Remember that rolling out the clay is hard work, so give a hand if you feel that the effort is becoming too much for your child, and that he or she may lose interest in the rest of the activity. When the clay is flat, the template is laid on the clay, and cut around with a wooden knife (see Figure 7.2). The tile is now complete and can be decorated by any method you and your child choose.

Try making texture patterns by pressing things into the clay. Try drawing on the clay by making scratch marks or adding pieces of clay and clay worm. Mix several methods and invent your own combinations.

Although the tiles have been cut to the size and shape of the template, don't be disappointed or dissatisfied if they become slightly misshapen when decorated. The idea of using a template is not intended to be a restriction, but a way of encouraging new skills and a more disciplined way of working. When the tiles are left to dry, make sure that they dry slowly and evenly. Try placing them on a cake cooling pan; sometimes it is a good idea to turn them over now and again, or put them under plastic to slow down the drying process. If clay is left to dry out unattended, even at room temperature, the edges will begin to curl up and become hard and brittle, long before the middle of the tile is dry.

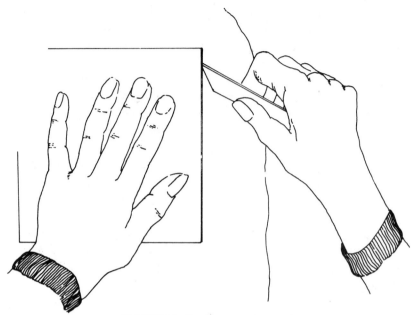

FIGURE 7.2. Cutting around a template.

Try making tiles cut around templates of different shapes, and experiment with your child in making and cutting clay shapes without using a template. These shapes will be odd, weird, and wonderful—but it is all good practice for your child in controlling movements and using the cutting knife.

SHAPED "PICTURE" TILES

As an alternative to simply drawing or painting an object or thing that interests your child, you can encourage him or her to draw in clay or to use a similar method to that described above, to make a tile picture. Clay can become another material with which to make pictures, just as it has been a material for making patterns. It is quite possible that a child will have begun using clay to make flat pictures through modeling and shaping clay in his or her hands. What I suggest here can be a way of encouraging that kind of work. Alternatively, it is a way of combining picture-making skills with the skills of physical control used in tile making.

Instead of using a square cardboard template, you cut the template for a shaped picture tile to the same shape as a drawing made by your child. The drawing can be of anything, and does not have to be complicated or sophisticated looking. It is impossible to suggest subject matter for this or any other work, but very simple ideas—a house, person, or animal—can be used for tile pictures. Remember that the best subject matter for your child will be what the child thinks of, and if nothing comes to mind, you are in a good position to suggest or help the child to remember things that you know he or she has found interesting. Make as much reference to things that you know have relevance to the child as possible. Use outings, holidays, the family, and pets as starting points.

Once the drawing is complete, get your child to cut around the main outline. The resulting shape can be used as a paper template, or it can be used as a pattern for cutting a cardboard template. Don't be concerned about distortions appearing in the drawing. What seem to be inaccuracies often reflect a child's feeling about what is important about the subject matter.

As before, the template has to be placed on the rolled clay and marked out and cut around with a wooden pottery knife. Decorate the tile with any mixture of techniques that seem suitable to the picture. Encourage your child to make positive choices about the appropriateness of the different methods.

USING CLAY FOR POTS

As clay is traditionally the material from which pots are made, it seems appropriate to include some potter's skills relevant to the level of development in this chapter. Should you wish more and fuller information about pottery techniques, consult a craft book or contact a practicing potter.

Making pots from solid lumps of clay.   For children who have made holes in a ball of clay with their thumb or finger and experimented squeezing the edges around the hole (Chapter 6), this idea is simply a refinement. This method needs good physical control and sustained interest. As the method is quite complicated, try it out yourself first to get the feel of it. Knowing what it feels like to make a shape in this way, and appreciating the difficulties, will help you to explain the method more easily. If you seek additional advice, this method is usually called making "thumb" or "pinch" pots.

Don't expect a high standard of finish, but attempt to get the idea of making a hollow shape established. Allow a child to use his or her own ideas about the final shape. Encourage your child to work with a lump of clay rolled or patted into a ball so that it fits comfortably into the hand, about the size of a tennis ball, or a little smaller.

Holding the ball of clay lightly in one hand, press a hole into the clay, reaching almost to the bottom, with a finger or thumb (Figure 7.3). Many children find it difficult to use their thumbs to begin with, but this method is best done with the thumb as it makes a larger hole. Still holding the clay lightly in one hand, put the thumb of the other hand back inside the clay, letting the fingers come around the outside of the ball. Gently squeeze thumb and fingers together, squeezing the "sides" of the pot. By moving the clay around the thumb, squeezing in the same way at every turn, the hole is gradually widened and the sides become more obvious. Finally, the sides can be modeled and squeezed into shape.

Flat clay made into pots.   Clay that has been rolled out evenly with the use of battens can be molded or curved into pots. Plaster of Paris molds either hollowed or domed can be bought to lay clay into or over. Other suitable molds can be improvised, as suggested later. Molds are easy to use, but should the following brief description be inadequate, consult a craft pottery book.

FIGURE 7.3. Making a hole in a ball of clay.

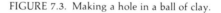

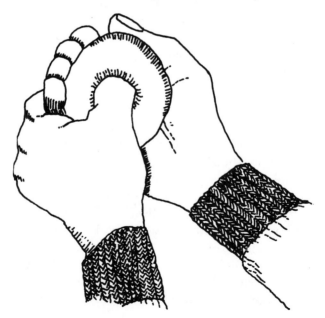

1. Trim the flattened clay to the right shape for the mold. Cut the shape a bit bigger than the mold, so that there is enough clay to stretch up to make the sides of the bowl. Encourage your child to judge the appropriate size, placing the mold on the clay as a guide.

2. Depending upon the type of mold (hollow or domed), lay the clay carefully onto, or over, the mold. The clay must be smoothed out to fit the mold completely, excluding all the air.

3. Next, trim the clay level with the edge of the mold. Encourage your child to use a wooden pottery knife to trim the clay, turning the mold as he or she works around.

4. Smooth the edges. Show your child how to smooth the cut edge with his or her fingers or a damp sponge.

As the clay dries, it will shrink away from the plaster mold and can then be lifted away as a complete bowl. Be particularly careful to remove clay formed over a dome-shaped mold as soon as it is dry enough to do so, because should the clay shrink too much, it will split over the mold.

Using the basic method, encourage your child to be as experimental and as expressive as possible. Avoid making the method so important that the fun of making pots is lost. Find other ways of making pots from flat clay. A simple but effective bowl can be made by cutting a shape in flat clay and supporting the edges of the shape on fat coils of clay, until dry. The coils of clay raise the edges, producing a shallow bowl shape. They can be discarded as soon as the clay is dry. Try making pots inside other bowls or saucers, but be careful to line them with canvas or other suitable material to stop the clay sticking. Experiment making pots over domes made from tightly packed newspaper balls or even stuffed paper bags!

Something to Talk About

The following game can be played in odd moments. Although it is best played with a small group of children, it can be played with only yourself and a child.

PICTURE CONSEQUENCES
Each person needs a strip of paper about 30 cm (12 in.) long and 10 cm (4 in.) wide—but it could be bigger. The idea is that a figure should be drawn, in sections, on these strips of paper; each player contributes a section.

Fold the paper into four equal sections, width wise. In the top section a head must be drawn, in the second a body to the waist, in the third the body and legs to the knees, and in the last section the rest of the legs and the feet. (If these divisions of the body seem too complex for your child, invent your own divisions. Try using only three sections, one for the head, one for the body, and the third for the legs and feet.)

The idea is that each complete picture should be drawn by four people. Each person has a strip of paper, and in the top section draws a head, and then passes the picture to someone else. Everyone should then receive a picture of a head, and on this they should draw, in the next section, a body to the waist, and then hand the paper on again. The rest of the body is added, and so on. This is more complex to explain than to do, but children need to play the game more than once to get the hang of it. It's a silly game, but can be fun to play. The comparison at the end can provoke interesting conversation. Children like to identify the part of a person that they drew, or sometimes make astute observations about their own and other contributions.

Once the game is established, it is even better if each section is folded over out of sight, except for tiny lines to indicate where the drawing is to be continued from, before handing on. The surprise at the end of the game is much greater when played in secret.

Children who have reached an advanced stage in their drawing may be able to make their drawing fit almost exactly the divisions on the paper, so that everyone draws a head of about the same size, a body and legs of the same size. It is then possible to make a "mix and match" book (see Figure 7.4). Staple all the pictures together along the left-hand side to form the pages of the book. Then cut each picture along the dividing fold lines, leaving about 1 cm (½ in.) uncut at the left-hand side of each division. Now the pages can be turned over in four separate sections, allowing the bodies to be mixed and matched at will.

This Is How I See It

As a child matures, his or her ability to remember things gets better, and it is quite natural for a child to make pictures about things that have happened to him or her.

I CAN REMEMBER

There is a kind of magic in a child being able to draw and make things that show what he or she can remember. It is exciting to see

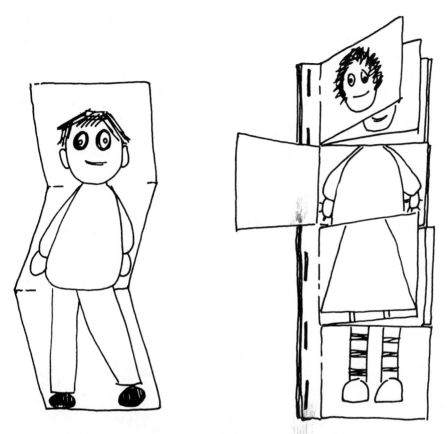

FIGURE 7.4. Picture consequences and a mix and match book.

what part of an experience a child remembers the best and wants to put into a picture. Many "out of school" activities prompt artwork—they add to the richness of a child's life, and it is rewarding to witness some of the impact that they make on him or her.

If your child shows an inclination to make drawings or paintings about things that have happened, or about things that he or she has done, encourage the child to recall those memories. Share your own memories, prompt your child to recall things he or she may have forgotten. Attempt to have available things like photographs, slides, and other information relating to places visited, as another way to help your child to remember and to stimulate a fresh look. If a picture is about an experience that you know was shared with a person other than yourself, try to make an opportunity for that person to respond to your child's work. All this is valuable sharing.

Encourage your child to choose his or her own materials for making a picture. Help him or her decide whether paints or crayons, pencils or felt pens will be the best things to use for a particular piece of work. The more often a child is encouraged to make a simple choice, the more able he or she will be to make spontaneous choices.

The communicative value of art activities such as these is increasingly great—and it is quite possible for children suffering profound language problems to learn to communicate a great deal through their pictures.

GO AND LOOK

As well as making pictures about things that have happened in the past, encourage your child to make pictures about things that her or she can see at the moment. If there is nothing in the art room that really catches the interest, go out and look elsewhere.

Find points of interest in the building in which you work, in the local area, or farther afield in a museum or zoo. Help your child to

FIGURE 7.5. This is how I see it—a monster made from a sketch done at a museum.

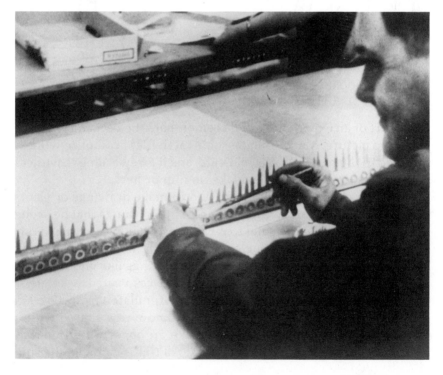

decide what he or she would like to look at, if possible, or at least share in advance any plans that you have in mind.

Work can relate to something that is already a point of interest in a school or club, to a focal point such as an aquarium, for instance. Work on something in the immediate locality can grow from expressed interests or conversation, but, of course, this relies on a familiarity with the outside. Museum visits can be either arranged with the intention of stimulating new ideas (see Figure 7.5), or as a followup to other work.

When working away from home or classroom, make life as easy as possible. Make a simple clipboard by clipping a sheet of paper onto a piece of stiff cardboard with a big clip (see Figure 7.6). This provides a firm surface to lean on, and the paper is held firmly and won't move around. Although it is too difficult to paint on the spot, colored crayons or felt pens can provide the necessary color.

Once the drawings have been made on the spot, they can be taken back into the art room and become the starting point for paintings, collage work, or work in clay. Remain flexible in the ways you encourage children to interpret their ideas, making use of all the techniques that they have learned.

MATERIALS

As your child progresses through the activities suggested in this book, you will find little need to buy different additional materials. Here are some you may like to add to your collection.

Paints.   Make sure you have a good selection of colors available at this stage. As a child's awareness increases, he or she will want more and more colors to choose from.

Brushes.   Introduce some smaller brushes to your collection to give your child a greater variety to the kinds of marks that can be made.

Drawing materials.   Pencil crayons may be a useful addition at this stage. They are almost like a pencil to work with, and they make a fairly fine line, so they can also be used to make fairly controlled drawings. They can be used to color in quite large areas as well.

Paper.   Continue to have colored paper available, if possible. The background color for drawings and paintings will probably become more important to your child as he or she progresses through the suggestions. Even if this does not become apparent, offer a choice on some occasions.

Scissors. At this stage most children will be able to begin to use scissors. Your child may not find small scissors the most easy to use, so be prepared to experiment and find the size most comfortable for him or her.

FIGURE 7.6. A clipboard.

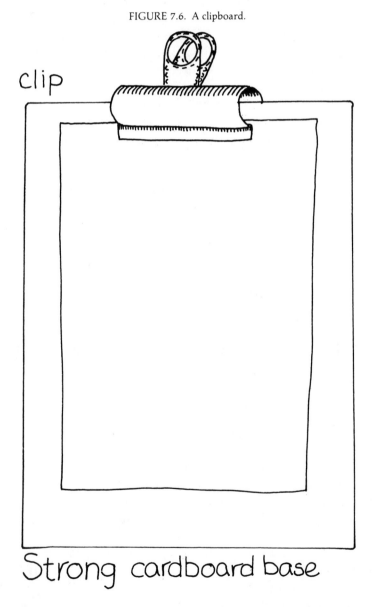

clip

Strong cardboard base

Cardboard.   Scraps of cardboard are essential for making templates for pottery work. The backs of writing pads may do.

Collage and "junk" materials.   It is of increasing value to have an odd assortment of materials available. Some of these may be other people's junk. Collect things you think will be useful. Some things may not have a use for some time, but if you have space to store it, continue your collection.

Clipboard.   Make a clipboard from strong cardboard and a big clip (see Figure 7.6).

Pottery tools.   Although they are not essential, you may like to collect some wooden pottery tools, useful for shaping and smoothing the clay. Not only do these tools have a practical use, but in using them your child is getting valuable practice in controlling small tools.

Scraper.   Metal and rubber scrapers, to smooth the surface of clay pieces, can begin to be of use at this stage.

8

Activities for Stage 6

STAGE 6: SEEING, KNOWING, AND MAKING

This chapter on activities for stage 6 is the final one on "things to do" in this book. Much of the work suggested is closely related to work suggested in previous chapters. Most suggestions rely on a child's familiarity with materials. Some understanding as to what different materials can be made to do is essential. At this stage, activities rely on good physical dexterity and discriminative powers. A child will probably have a fairly clear idea of what he or she wants to do before beginning, and be able to organize the basic materials and equipment he or she will need for an activity.

The activities in this chapter are designed to encourage careful observation and thought about how best to make a particular piece of work. They are intended to encourage a child to organize him- or herself with sufficient forethought to be able to achieve what he or she has set out to do.

There are fewer practical suggestions in this section because it becomes increasingly inappropriate to suggest specific activities. Most of the suggestions relate as much to an attitude as to a method, with the exception of those relating to clay work, which include some more technical hints. Try reading all the suggestions in this chapter to see how they relate to your situation and your child before beginning. Do not be put off by the lack of specific activities, as both you and your child will have developed your own ideas about ways of working with materials and will have ideas on what to do next.

GENERAL HINTS

MAKE MATERIALS AVAILABLE

Try to make a selection of materials available to your child so that he or she can make the choice and begin to organize his or her own activities. Try to be flexible in your approach to art activities, so that, should your child want to use certain materials in particular, there is at least sometimes freedom to do so. Don't forget that even children who have apparently lost interest in certain kinds of materials may have their interest reawakened at any time. Be prepared to reintroduce materials that have been ignored for a time.

ORGANIZING EQUIPMENT

Whenever it is practical, encourage your child to choose the materials and equipment required for a particular piece of work. Keep as many materials as you can in easily accessible places, perhaps leaving some visible on open shelves. As far as possible, always store things in the same place.

When planning an activity, help your child to think what he or she is going to need, so that the child anticipates needs before beginning. This can be done by talking about what the child is going to do, and about how he or she is going to do it. As always, be sensitive to your child's stage of learning, and give directions and even help when really necessary. But remember, just because it takes longer for your child to organize things than it does for you to do it is no reason to offer help. As long as the child is happy to do things for him- or herself, give encouragement and enough time to get it done at the child's own pace.

SELF-MOTIVATED WORK

At this stage a child will have an increased awareness of what he or she can do, and will be sufficiently familiar with materials and methods of work to be able to make things by him- or herself. A child will be able to decide not only what to do, but also how he or she is going to do it. Encourage your child to explore his or her own ideas—they are just as good as any you or I may have, and this step toward independent work is very important in development.

FINDING A SOLUTION

Try to help your child to solve problems for him- or herself. As always, your observations are very important to your understanding of your child and his or her work. Be aware of what the child is doing, and how he or she goes about doing and making things. Should the child have difficulties making things go as wanted, attempt to help solve the problems, if you can, rather than do it for him or her. Making things as easy for your child as you can, try to lead the child to find his or her own solution to a problem. Help the child to think about what needs to be done next to make it "right"; perhaps offer a forgotten tool, a clue, or a suggestion as to what he or she might try. Give help and support, without taking over.

A FREEDOM TO EXPLORE

As at any other stage of development, children need opportunities to explore and experiment with materials, to discover more and more about the possibilities available to them. This kind of exploration can lead to positive learning at all stages, so allow your child time just to play with materials. Do not be worried if there is nothing to show as an immediate result of such free activity.

WHAT I CAN DO—
AND WHAT I CANNOT

As a child's general awareness grows, he or she will inevitably become more aware of what he or she is able and, conversely, unable to do. An awareness of ability to do things can be very satisfying and can build self-confidence, but an awareness of inabilities can be unsettling. Should the awareness of inabilities become acute, a child may feel unhappy or frustrated. It can be frustrating for anyone to be unable to do the things that they want to do—yet if kept in perspective, one's abilities and inabilities can remain in balance without detriment to development. To maintain the balance requires a recognition of the value of one's abilities, so continue to show your regard for your child's work.

Although children cannot, and should not, be sheltered from work that has qualities that they would be unable to attain, do make it clear to your child that his or her work is of particular value, because it is done by that child. To avoid confusion, I rarely show work completed by another child as an example to follow, and suggest that any work used to illustrate a particular method should be very carefully selected. Present it in such a way that it does not appear as an ideal to achieve or an example of excellence to copy.

ART AND RELAXATION

Children may find that using art materials can be a relaxing experience and wish to use them differently for relaxation than when more positively intending to make something. Many adults respond in a similar way. Some simply enjoy handling clay without caring what they make; modeling whatever comes to mind. Others make nonsensical doodles just for fun. Respect your child's desire to use materials for personal relaxation, and don't make the child feel that he or she always has to make something to gain your respect.

THINGS TO DO

This Is How I See It

As in the previous chapter, much of the work here will be about things that have been seen and are remembered. More work than before will be about looking at things that can still be seen.

THINGS I REMEMBER

Continue to encourage your child to use the memory of things that have happened as a basis for artwork. Help the child to remember things seen, or things done, by sharing your memories. Remember that words describing something cannot replace a memory of what it looked like, and that sometimes photographs taken, or drawings made, on the spot may prove more help. Don't suggest that your child copy photographs, but use them as a reference to help remember details that he or she finds important and wants to remember more about (Figure 8.1). The things that a child chooses to leave out in a piece of work are just as important as the things chosen to include. The emphasis on some things, and lack of detail in others, is revealing.

Sometimes your child may find it useful or fun to make two pictures of the same thing. The first picture of a pair can often act as a way of stimulating memory and enable a child to remember even more than before. With the first picture seen as a kind of rehearsal, the second picture can then contain more memories and be done with a different kind of care. Both pieces of work are important.

Remind your child of the variety of materials available. If your child has made a picture in which he or she has remembered a number of different things, it can be useful to discuss alternative ways he or she could proceed. Some pictures lend themselves to

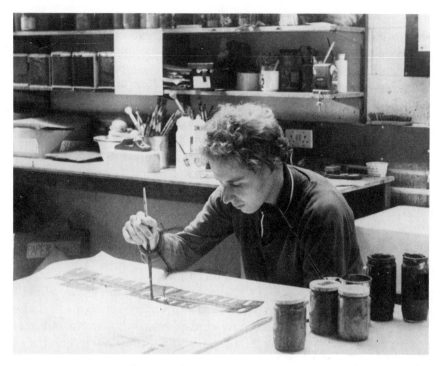

FIGURE 8.1. I can remember—a castle seen on vacation.

being made in blocks of color cut from paper or fabrics; others from a mixture of painting, with details drawn on top; yet others could be made from a combination of collage and drawing. Increasingly your child can be made aware of the different qualities of objects, and translate these into pictures. He or she may, for example, be able to choose materials that will best describe the hard rugged quality of a wall built of stone, or the soft flowing quality of water. Be flexible in your approach to materials, and encourage your child to find the best way he or she can think of for making a particular piece of work.

THINGS I CAN SEE

Making pictures about things that can be seen is a similar process to making things from memory, except that memory does not play a part in the choice of what is important and what is not. When making pictures about things that are remembered, the things that were not important are forgotten, and thus excluded from the pictures. It may be more difficult for a child to make pictures of things he or she *can* see, because the child may be less able to choose what is important and may want to put all the things he or she notices into one picture. The child may then encounter difficulties in getting the picture to look "right" and want to know how to do it right. There is, of course, no one way of making a picture "right": each person will make a different picture from the next, and all of them will be "right."

Attempt to help your child to describe what it is he or she is trying to put into the work, and thus help the child to decide what it is that he or she finds most important (see Figure 8.2). Sometimes the child may be most concerned with the shapes he or she can see, or the colors, or perhaps the texture. Whatever the child chooses to emphasize is right for that child, so help to find the best materials and the best way he or she can make the picture "right."

FINDING OUT ABOUT IT

It is likely that at some time children at this stage will be motivated to do work about things of which they have only a small amount of experience. They may want to prepare work for a particular occasion, which requires some kind of research into the subject. For instance, when making a flag to fly on a camping trip, children I

FIGURE 8.2. I know—looking and drawing.

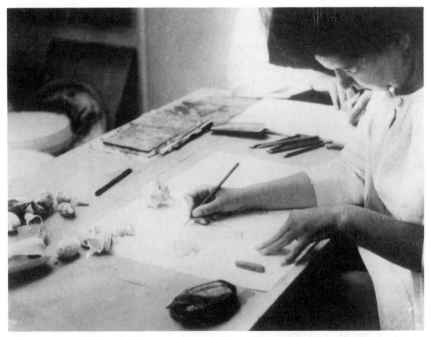

taught had to think about and find a suitable design. Having found a design that they thought might be suitable, they had to go to a library and find out what it stood for, to see if it really was suitable.

When organizing children to work in a group, it can be of value to help them to find a task that involves them in some modest research, so that each person has to find something out about the subject, and so has something special to contribute to the joint effort. Research may mean simply going to have another look at something, but may mean going to ask someone else for help, or to find some extra information, perhaps from books.

LOOKING FOR DETAIL

As a child's awareness becomes sharper, he or she will be able to see more detail in things. Doing artwork can encourage close observation and will in turn help to develop powers of discrimination. On some occasions encourage your child to pay particular attention to aspects of detail in his or her own work. Be sensitive in your comments, so that without appearing critical you are able to lead your child to take a little extra care in the way he or she looks at things, or in the way he or she works.

FINDING A PATTERN

When children have the ability to look at things and to make some record of what they can see, patterns and designs can be discovered in all kinds of different things. Patterns can be fun to discover. Remade in different materials, they can be used as a basis for decorative collages or designs made in clay, or they can be recreated as drawings or paintings.

FLOATING PATTERNS

Unpredictable patterns can be made by floating oil paint, household oil-based paint, or drawing inks on water. Line a bowl with plastic to prevent the oil paint from staining it. A plastic shopping bag could be cut to fit a mixing bowl, but sheet plastic will probably be necessary to line other bowls.

Fill the bowl with water and drop a little paint or ink into the water. As water and oil will not mix, the paint should rise to the top and float on the water. To pick up the resulting pattern, drop a piece of fairly absorbent paper onto the water, and it will soak up the paint. Ordinary white drawing paper or writing paper should be all right to use; experiment with different sorts and compare the results. Pick the paper off the water and leave it to dry with the painty side up. The paper must be handled with care as the paint will remain wet for a little while and must be dried out completely before further work can be done.

Encourage your child to experiment mixing the color on the water. He or she can use an old skewer or piece of stick to move the water slightly to make the colors swirl and mix together (see Figure 8.3).

BLOT PATTERNS

Blot patterns are made by putting a blot of paint or ink onto a fairly smooth paper, and then folding the paper in half. As the paper is folded, the paint is squashed between the two halves of the paper and spreads out to leave a mirrored pattern when the paper is opened out again. Experiment with various types of paper. If the paper is too absorbent the paint will not spread out so much, and the pattern made will be less interesting.

Patterns can be made on quite small pieces of paper, applying

FIGURE 8.3. Finding the floating pattern.

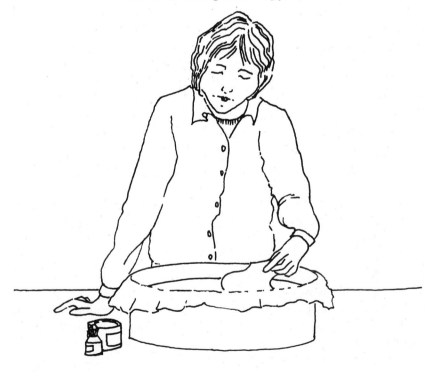

the paint with a small brush or squeezing ink from a fountain pen. On larger paper, try applying the paint from a slip trailer (or squeezy bottle), or daubing it on with large brushes or sponges.

Open out the pattern and enjoy the surprise. Encourage your child to experiment making different effects according to where he or she put a color before folding the paper in half. Try using two or three colors that go together well, and see how they mix after the paper is folded.

EXPLORING A PATTERN

Patterns are made of mixtures of different colors and arrangements of lines and shapes. When doing work based on a pattern, it is useful to decide which particular quality is the most interesting to explore.

Patterns in which colored shapes are most interesting may best be recreated in blocks of colored paper torn or cut to shape, or painted in bold colored areas. Paper collage is a flexible method of work in which several different colors can be placed on top of one another, and shapes can easily be altered or adjusted. (When looking at blot patterns, explore the possibility of folding the collage paper in half and then cutting or tearing from it shapes based on one half of the blot pattern. When the collage sheet is opened, it will have two mirrored halves just like the blot pattern.) Patterns in which line is most important are best remade in materials with their own linear qualities, such as pencils, crayons, or delicate painting.

Clay can be used to make patterns based on shapes or lines. Begin with a piece of clay rolled flat as a base, then use clay worms to make the lines in the pattern. Shapes can either be drawn onto the clay, or cut from flat clay and attached using the usual method. Scratch the surfaces to be joined, apply some slip, and press the two pieces together. This kind of pattern can be used as a decoration on a pot.

Getting the Desired Result

Having reached this stage of development, your child will be able to complete tasks involving a number of different processes. He or she will be able to remember several steps that make up a complete process, but don't forget that the child will need your help to begin with in remembering all the steps.

Several of the skills required for more sophisticated methods of making pots have already been learned by your child. Complex methods can be made easier if broken down into a number of known skills, to be done in the correct order.

SLAB POTS

It is beyond the scope of this book to give detailed instructions on how to make the rectangular slab pots, but a breakdown of the skills required is as follows:

1. Rolling out clay between battens.
2. Cutting around templates; four required for the sides, one for the base.
3. Joining the sides together by scratching and applying slip; try marking the templates to indicate which surfaces are to be joined together.
4. Joining the base to the sides by scratching and applying slip. Get help from a craft book or from a practical potter before attempting this method—and be sure that you understand the method before introducing it to your child.

MAKING CYLINDERS
FROM FLAT CLAY

Slabs of flat clay can be fairly easily molded into round cylinders. These can be made into pots by adding a base, but try using long thin tubes as a base for figures! Try your own variations.

Roll a piece of clay flat between battens. The clay is going to be wrapped around a cylindrical form such as a can, so make the clay long enough to go around the can, perhaps 15–20 cm (6–8 in.) wide to begin with. Trim the width of the clay to size, and trim one end straight.

Although it is best to use a wooden cylindrical form, and a rolling pin will do, a shorter, fatter form is easier to use, about the size of a soup can.

Wrap newspaper around the can and tape it down with masking tape. This is done so that the clay will not stick to the can. Lay the can on the clay, and roll the clay around it. When the two ends of the clay meet around the can, leave enough overlap to make a seam and trim all the extra clay off. Join the clay by pinching the two edges together, making a seam that sticks out all the way down the cylinder (see Figure 8.4).

Stand the cylinder on end, and either add a base or leave as an open-ended tube.

To add a base, place the tube on a piece of flattened clay. Draw

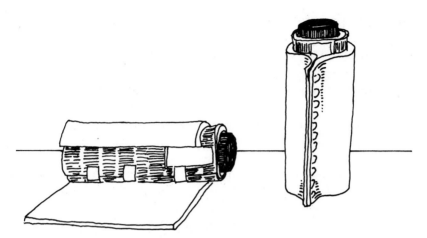

FIGURE 8.4. Making and creating from a clay tube.

around the base and cut out the shape with a pottery knife. Scratch the edges to be joined and seal with slip.

Apart from helping your child to learn the method by getting each step completed in the correct order, help him or her to use and refine the cylinder to become something else. Make a tall pot decorated by scratching a pattern onto it—by pressing textures onto it, drawing with clay worms, or even cutting pieces out of the sides. Transform it into a figure by adding a head and arms, or lay flat to form the body of a monster animal.

OTHER POTTERY METHODS

Some children at this stage will be able to learn how to make coil pots without difficulty, and some may even be able to use a potter's wheel. Neither method is described here, as they are complicated to describe and much better learned by watching someone else and copying—or having one's hands directed by an expert.

There is no particular value to a child in learning complex technical processes, unless he or she has a particular interest in that direction. In that case, contact a local community center or evening school. As with all the work described in the book, the value has to be in what it does for your child—how it helps to develop either skills or personality. Never allow a process to become a restriction, by insisting that it be done exactly right, when the child is not ready for such rigor.

MATERIALS

The materials used in this chapter are mostly those already used in previous sections. Many of the activities rely on a child's familiarity with materials, so make a good selection available.

Paints. Poster colors and ready-mix paints offer good strong clear colors.

Brushes. Have a good range of brushes of different shapes and sizes available.

Drawing materials. Have a selection of different drawing materials available. Wax crayons, oil pastels, and felt pens make clear bright colors. Pencils of different weights, ball point pens, and felt markers are good for making line drawings, and there is a wide range of other drawing pens on the market, some of which are quite cheap. Pencil crayons can be used to make fine lines or to block in areas of color.

Paper. Continue to make available paper of various colors and texture. Try to offer a choice between large sheet or small.

Collage materials. If it has proved possible, continue to collect interesting materials suitable for collage, both paper and fabric.

Drawing inks. Use drawing inks or oil-based paints for "floating patterns." To use drawing inks for picture making, buy "dip-in" pens.

Pottery tools. New tools are not a necessary addition, but they may prove useful and fun to use.

III
CONCLUSION

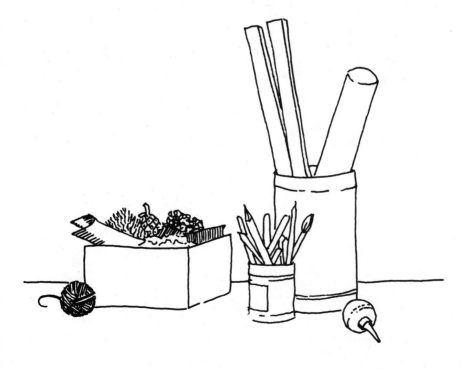

9
The End
Is Just a Beginning

Throughout the practical suggestions in this book, I have described how activities can be encouraged by breaking them down into simple steps, and how they can be useful to the development of skills and perception. But each activity, however simple, has a special value that can contribute toward a child's broader understanding of him- or herself and be a valuable means of self-expression.

Drawing, painting, and modeling can all be used as a way of showing what we find interesting, what we enjoy or find important. For some people, and children in particular, it is a natural way of sharing things with other people. Through art activities, they may be able to "get more across" than in words. The same can be true for a mentally handicapped person.

Remember that whatever level your child has reached, the help offered in this book is only a beginning. As soon as your child has some simple skills and is able to use materials, he or she has a valuable means of expression that you can help him or her to use best. Using this book as a guide, find ways of helping your child to develop work and ideas, and thus explore his or her potential to the fullest.

IT'S NOT AS EASY AS IT SEEMS

I have tried in this book to be as practical and straightforward as possible, to be realistic about the provision of activities and in the approach to activities. All the ideas contained here are based on personal teaching experience. Providing art activities for either individuals or groups of people is not easy. To begin with it may be difficult because equipment and space are inadequate, but it is made far more difficult because each person that you work with will have a different reaction to the activities you provide. In this chapter, let us share some of the problems I have met and discuss the ways I attempted (not always successfully) to solve them.

The problems seem to fall into three categories: those related to additional physical difficulties suffered by a child; those related to a child's inability to communicate with words; and the most upsetting—those having to do with rejection of the activity, producing stubbornness and anger in a child.

MAKE IT AS EASY AS POSSIBLE

When a child is unable to do something because of a physical disability, it is often possible to adapt the activity to suit the individual needs. For a young man confined to a wheelchair with weakening arm and hand muscles, we were able to adapt a fitting on his wheelchair to take a reasonably large table. Since he did not have to stretch out far or lift his arms very much, he was able to use clay, paints, and crayons at his own fitted table. When his muscles became inevitably weaker, playdough replaced clay; it is softer material more easily manipulated. When it became difficult even to lift a brush into a paint can, he used wax crayons and felt pens.

Among several people suffering partial spastic paralysis, I found that art activities could help some and hinder others. Two students illustrate this. For one it was a joy to be able to make things, even though he did so very crudely to begin with. It was an exciting challenge to work hard to get things better. This concentrated hard work seemed to help him in other areas of development. For the other, whose efforts were equally great, the activities caused frustration and upset. It is possible that I did not encourage the most suitable art activities for this girl, but she was able to see and understand far more than she was physically able to do. She wanted to do more and became annoyed and frustrated because things would not "go right." In this case, praise and encouragement were not enough, and other activities, where she was able to keep up with her friends, proved to be much more fulfilling.

DO YOU UNDERSTAND?

Most of us are aware that we need to use words to tell people about things, and we are usually understood when we use words. For a child who does not speak well, or who cannot speak at all, life is made more complex. Earlier in this book I suggested that drawing and painting can offer such children an alternative way to telling us things. But how do we cope with a young person who obviously enjoys painting (or other art activity), yet does not make pictures of things and at the same time does very much want a response from us?

A boy I worked with was rather aggressive in his insistence on painting. He was happy to paint on the floor or at a table, and seemed content to use the colors provided—sometimes working in only one color. He understood about washing his brushes and about clearing up at the end of an activity. He did not want help or encouragement to make his paintings, often shaking his fist if interrupted, but he always came to get me to look at his completed paintings, tugging at my sleeve and grunting. I responded through visible actions and by talking. I attempted to communicate my pleasure and delight by smiling and generally admiring the work, but found it necessary to look at the painting carefully, pointing to various parts and talking about them. I have no idea how helpful this was. The child's speech did not develop noticeably and his paintings did not alter substantially. But he did continue to enjoy the activity and to demand my attention.

THIS IS NOT FOR ME

I have known several people who seem to be saying, by the way they behave, that art activities are not for them. I have had people break or tear things, people who shout, cry, or bite, and those who deliberately do silly things you would prefer them not to do. I believe these kinds of reactions arise for many different reasons. Some reactions seem to be a kind of showing off; others seem to indicate frustration; others stubbornness; and yet others a more deep-rooted disturbance.

One of my pupils sometimes deliberately drank the paint or paint water, or made very small tears in her own or others' paper. She always seemed to be looking to see if I was watching, and I believe she was hoping I would notice and give her my attention by telling her off. I attempted to ignore these things or to treat them in a matter-of-fact way, but I did not make much of them, wishing to give attention for good behavior, not bad. This became more difficult when she tore someone else's paper because I consider this totally unacceptable. The other person also got upset, thus drawing attention to her. Only occasionally did she make or draw anything herself, and then in a "throw away" manner. It was difficult to praise these as she seemed to find praise difficult to accept. I do not know whether I helped this girl, but I would still work on the principle that she should be praised for doing something constructive and creative, but should not get attention for doing harm. Had she done things that really harmed herself or others, however, I would have had to adopt a different attitude and found a way of restraining her.

Frustration can be the cause of antisocial behavior. It is a very intense feeling, and without a means to communicate it, the feeling can get out of hand. Many ordinary people throw things, hit people, and behave in a generally destructive way when frustrated, but I don't believe the choice for anyone should be limited to one between succeeding and disrupting a situation. Frustration can be caused by an awareness of one's own inabilities, by a feeling of failure. It is frustrating for anyone to be unable to achieve what they set out to do, so it is important to organize activities in which children can function at their own level. In particular, avoid using other children's work as demonstration pieces—it may prove more harmful than helpful—unless you are confident that your child can make something he or she will recognize as being as good as the example.

In some cases the stimulation of art activities seems to produce undesirable effects, as though the activities are disturbing. I worked with a girl who was happy drawing rather intense colored patterns, but she resented interruption, sometimes pulling my hair when I spoke to her. This kind of thing is impossible to ignore, but I felt it possible to help with care. Unfortunately, the girl's behavior became worse. She turned over furniture and spoiled other people's work. As she was unable to talk and so to tell us what she felt, we eventually had to exclude her from the room because the atmosphere or the activities appeared to disturb her.

Art activities do not give pleasure to everyone, nor do they become important to everyone. As with any other activities, there will be those who choose to be excluded for some or all of the time. Never insist that anyone participate—but give as much encouragement and support, sensitive guidance, and firm care as possible to those who find them fulfilling or simply enjoyable.

IV

APPENDIXES

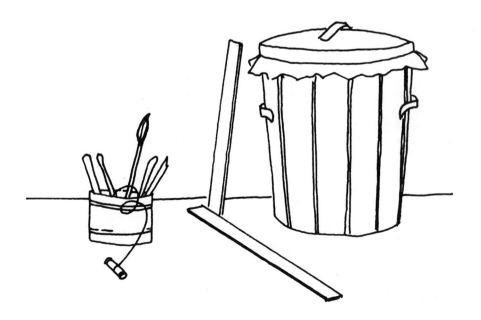

Appendix A: Introduction to the Use and Care of Clay

A separate introduction to the use of clay is included because, unlike most of the other materials mentioned in this book, clay is a specialist material. There are things about the storage and presentation of clay that need to be understood to ensure successful use. Don't be put off using clay—the following technical hints are all quite simple and can be learned and accommodated fairly easily, given enough space and a little planning.

WHY USE CLAY?

All children enjoy materials that can be handled, and those that can be squeezed, squashed, and made into different shapes have their own special magic. There are many different materials that have these properties, such as plasticine, playdough, cold clay, as well as clay. All these materials vary in their qualities and have various advantages and disadvantages, but of them all, clay seems the most satisfactory and rewarding to use.

WHAT ARE THE ALTERNATIVES?

Plasticine is a rather stiff material to handle, so it requires considerable strength to squeeze it. It is difficult to use in very large pieces and does not stick to itself very easily. (If you want to use plasticine and find it very hard, warmth will help to soften it, so leave it near a radiator or fire before use.)

Playdough is a very cheap way of providing a pliable material for children. It is made from equal quantities of flour and salt mixed to a dough with water and a little oil. Playdough can easily be stored in a plastic bag in the refrigerator for several days, and can be colored with food dyes without harm to the children. Although playdough is an extremely useful material, particularly in the early stages of development, it has little strength and can only be used to make things that will be supported on a flat surface.

Cold clay is a commercially produced clay that dries hard without baking, but is not brittle as ordinary clay would be before baking. Unfortunately, cold clay has a tendency to crumble when manipulated, which makes work difficult.

Clay is usually bought commercially in a cleaned and refined form. It is a very satisfactory material to handle as it is very easy to mold, and it can be modeled in large pieces or very delicately. Several pieces can be joined together firmly, and it has considerable strength even in its plastic state. Clay must be stored damp in airtight containers and ideally requires baking. The real disadvantage is the need for a kiln to bake the clay, which means a length of time between the making of an object and the end of the firing process.

WHAT KIND OF CLAY?

There are various different kinds of clay specially prepared for different uses, but the most basic kinds are either earthenware or stoneware. Earthenware is usually brown and stoneware is usually a pale stone color, but there is also brown stoneware and a pale gray earthenware clay.

When buying a clay, contact your local suppliers and ask their advice. Bear in mind the following points:

- A child may be reluctant to handle the brown clay as it seems dirty, so a pale clay is best to start with.
- If you consider adding a brown clay later, it is useful for both clays to bake at the same temperature.

TECHNICAL HINTS FOR PARENTS

How to store clay.   Clay is usually supplied soft and ready for use in large plastic bags. It can be stored in these bags for a considerable length of time, provided that the bag is not damaged in any way. It is essential that the water in the clay does not evaporate. When clay is taken from the bag, either the remainder can be stored in an airtight container or the bag can be resealed. Plastic containers make ideal storage places for large quantities of clay. Even in airtight boxes, the clay should be covered with damp sacking cloth to prevent it from drying out.

Joining clay pieces together.   Just as two plasticine pieces can be pushed together to make a new shape, so too can clay pieces in the early stages. This is not always satisfactory, however, because the two pieces may not join together well. This kind of joining requires firm handling, so it may be necessary to assist your child by simply giving the clay pieces a final "push" together.

A more permanent and satisfactory join can be made by scratching the two surfaces to be joined and damping them with water or slip. (Slip is dry powder clay mixed with water to a thick but runny consistency; see below.)

Don't discourage your child by insisting he or she attempt to use this second method before the child is ready to learn such a complex technique, but try to avoid the inevitable disappointments caused when clay pieces fall apart because the joints were badly made. It is possible to test joints for weakness after a child has finished work and to rejoin those that are badly made yourself.

How to make a slip.   Slip is powdered clay mixed with water to a thick but runny consistency. To make a slip, allow some clay to dry out completely and grind it into a fairly fine powder. Break large pieces by hitting them with a mallet or rolling pin, then crush them small under a rolling pin. Put the powder into a container and gradually mix with a little water. Add enough water to form a thick but runny paste; store in an airtight container, perhaps a food container of plastic with close fitting lid.

To make different colored slips, a powder oxide can be added to the runny mixture. For details and advice on which oxide to add and how much, contact your supplier.

How to reclaim dry clay.   Clay can dry out and become too brittle to use, but as long as it has not been fired, it can always be reclaimed for use later.

If the clay has dried out only a little, but has become too brittle to model easily, make the clay into a ball shape, push a hole into the center with your finger, fill it with water, and seal the hole. The clay may need kneading to distribute the water, or it may absorb it fairly well in a short time without help.

If the clay has become completely dry and brittle, it must be broken into small pieces and allowed gradually to reabsorb water. This requires a second container, although for small quantities an ice cream carton from the freezer may be large enough. First, break large lumps of clay with something heavy like a mallet. Break the brittle clay into small pieces, then crush even smaller with a rolling pin. To prevent small pieces or dust flying all over the place, cover the clay with sacking or other coarse cloth before beginning to roll it. Cover the bottom of the container with the small clay pieces and then squirt water on it until it is completely wet. The idea is to allow the clay to reabsorb enough water to make it plastic again, but not so much that it becomes slush. I use an old dishwashing liquid bottle to squirt the water onto the dry clay. When the first layer of clay is wet, add a second layer of dry clay and wet that too. Continue adding thin layers of dry clay, each wetted in turn, until all the clay is used up. Place a damp cloth on top. It may be necessary to add more water later, and as it cannot be added to the bottom layer, holes must be made through the clay with a stick and water poured into them. Leave the clay until it has absorbed enough water to be wetter than the clay ready to use; it should be on the sticky side.

The sticky clay should now be turned out onto a table or dry plaster block. While it is drying, clay should be turned to dry all surfaces and wedged to get rid of trapped air. Gradually, the extra water will dry out and the clay will revert to a soft workable consistency.

When working, never leave any clay uncovered for a long time. If taking a break, cover the clay work with a damp cloth.

Coloring clay. The traditional way to finish clay work is to apply a glaze, which can be colored or transparent, glossy or matte. But there are other alternatives, such as using oxides or color stains under clear glaze.

Although glazing pottery can be a fairly simple process, it needs some skill in application. A basic transparent glaze can be mixed from a tested recipe and colored with the addition of a small percentage of metal oxides. The clay suppliers will probably have a reliable basic glaze recipe and will recommend the temperature at which it matures. Seek professional advice on application (dipping, pouring, and spraying) either from the suppliers or from a craft book concerned with basic clay work.

One of the greatest problems concerning the coloring of clay is that a rare glaze is white or only slightly colored when applied to the pottery, and so gives no indication of the color it will be after the second firing. For many children this breaks the continuity of the work, and they have difficulty recognizing their own work after the second firing. These difficulties introduce an apparently random and unsatisfactory element to the work.

Color stains can partially solve the problem. Color stains come in powder form that can be applied to pottery when mixed with water. They can be applied with a brush and remain the same color throughout the glaze firing; thus children are able to retain the identity of their work. As the stain contains no glaze, a transparent glaze has to be used on top. This is, of course, opaque white before firing and covers the stains completely. So that a child could retain memory of the colors used on a piece of work, you might apply the glaze yourself, just before firing. Only after introducing and demonstrating the idea that pottery goes into the kiln white and comes out colored did I suggest that a child complete the coloring process him- or herself.

Baking clay.   All clay needs baking at least once after it has dried out completely, to make it more durable and solid. And objects that are to be finished with a glaze will need baking twice. The first baking is known as a greenware firing, the second as a glazing firing. Clay has to be baked in a special oven, known as a kiln, in which the temperatures reached are much higher than in a domestic oven.

THE KILN

Getting a kiln, or access to a kiln.   If you are fortunate enough to be able to acquire a pottery kiln of your own, it is advisable to contact various suppliers and discuss the most suitable model for your particular situation and requirements. Describe where the kiln is to be placed and the sort of work you will be firing, and explain how often you anticipate using the kiln. As the temperature inside a kiln is much greater than inside a domestic oven and the weight of the fire bricks lining the chamber is considerable, care must be taken in the placing of a kiln and in the provision of ventilation. Like the domestic oven, kilns need a high electrical voltage and, unless they are very small "test" kilns, cannot be plugged into an ordinary socket.

Most parents and many educational or social establishments will not be able to afford to buy, or have suitable space to accommodate, a kiln of their own, but someone else may be willing to fire work for you. Local independent potters or potters working in potteries attached to suppliers may be willing to fire complete or part loads for you. Or you may be able to make an arrangement with a local or evening school with a pottery kiln to fire work for you.

Packing and firing clay work.   Pieces of unglazed pottery can be packed close together, or even stacked inside one another. It does not matter if unglazed pottery touches another unglazed piece. But glazed pottery must not come into contact with other pottery or with the sides of the kiln. For both firings, space must be left around the work to allow the hot air to circulate. For more detailed advice and details regarding temperatures and such, contact the suppliers of the clay and the kiln, but remember that just as every domestic oven is slightly different from another, so too is a kiln, and best results are achieved with experience.

PRESENTATION OF CLAY WORK

Most clay work, free-standing modeled pieces or pots, need no additional display, for they stand as finished pieces in their own right, but sometimes flat pottery pieces benefit from special display. Particularly when flat pottery pieces are like pictures drawn in or with clay, it may seem appropriate to mount them so that they can be hung on the wall like a picture. The weight of clay requires that it be mounted on fairly substantial board—plywood works well. To make a pleasant but neutral background, stretch burlap around the board before mounting the pottery. Use a strong polyvinyl, acrylic-based glue to stick the pottery to the board.

BASIC EQUIPMENT

Clay.   White, stoneware or earthenware, and/or brown earthenware. If using two clays, choose them to fire at the same temperature.

Two storage containers.   Both must be airtight. One is for the clay ready for use and could be a strong plastic bag; the second is for clay being "reclaimed" after having become too dry and could be an ice cream carton. For large quantities, plastic boxes are ideal.

Sacking.   To be placed damp on top of clay being stored.

Empty dishwashing liquid bottle.   To be filled with water for the reclaiming process.
  For other materials and equipment, see the list of materials at the end of Chapters 5, 6, 7, and 8.

Appendix B: Supplier and Craft Information

SUPPLIERS

Most large towns have art and craft shops or department stores that will sell or order most of the materials suggested in this book. College or university bookstores will also stock or will order supplies listed here. Art supply stores will usually be able to tell you all you need to know about finding appropriate materials for any art activities mentioned in these chapters. For supplies specifically designed for the handicapped, the following organizations may be helpful.

ABC School Supply, Inc.
6500 Peachtree Industrial Boulevard
Norcross, GA 30071

Amaco Art Supply
4717 W. 16th Street
Indianapolis, IN 46222

American Foundation for the Blind
Consumer Products Department
15 W. 16th Street
New York, NY 10011

Child Craft Education Corporation
Special Needs Division
20 Kilmer Road
Edison, NJ 08817

Developmental Learning Materials
#1 DLM Park
Allen, TX 75002

Edmark, Inc.
P.O. Box 3903
Bellevue, WA 98009

EDUCAT Publishers, Inc.
P.O. Box 2891
Clinton, IA 52735

Flaghouse, Inc.·
18 W. 18th Street
New York, NY 10011

Gamco Industries
Educational Materials for the Exceptional
Box 1862B
Big Spring, TX 79720

Key School Supply, Inc.
P.O. Box 351, 128 Zebulon Street
Barnesville, GA 30204

National School Products
114 W. Broadway
Maryville, TN 37801

Preston Corporation
Materials for Exceptional Children
71 Fifth Avenue
New York, NY 10003

Selected Materials for Special Students
Opportunities for Learning, Inc.
8950 Lurline Avenue, Dept. JK6
Chatsworth, CA 91311

Special Education Materials, Inc.
484 S. Broadway
Yonkers, NY 10705

CRAFT PUBLICATIONS

The following magazines may be helpful sources of information on supplies and activities.

Arts and Activities
Publishers Development Corporation
591 Camino de la Reina, Suite 200
San Diego, CA 92108

Ceramic Arts and Crafts
Scott Advertising Publishing Company
30595 W. Eight Mile Road
Livonia, MI 48152

Ceramics Monthly
Professional Publications Inc.
Box 12248, 1609 NW Boulevard
Columbus, OH 43212

Craft, Model and Hobby Industry
Hobby Publications Inc.
225 W. 34th Street
New York, NY 10001

Crafts Magazine
PJS Publications
News Plaza, Box 1790
Peoria, IL 61656

Crafts 'n Things
Clapper Publishing Co., Inc.
14 Main Street
Park Ridge, IL 60068

Creative Crafts
Carstens Publications Inc.
Box 700
Newton, NJ 07860

Index